O U L

OXFORD UROLOGY LIBRARY

Nocturia

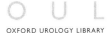

O U L
OXFORD UROLOGY LIBRARY

Nocturia

Edited by

Hashim Hashim

Consultant Urological Surgeon and Director of the Urodynamics Unit
Bristol Urological Institute
Southmead Hospital
Bristol, UK

Paul Abrams

Professor of Urology
Bristol Urological Institute
Southmead Hospital
Bristol, UK

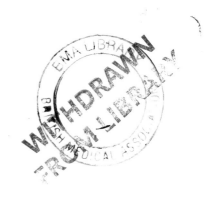

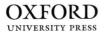

OXFORD
UNIVERSITY PRESS

OXFORD
UNIVERSITY PRESS

Great Clarendon Street, Oxford, OX2 6DP,
United Kingdom

Oxford University Press is a department of the University of Oxford.
It furthers the University's objective of excellence in research, scholarship,
and education by publishing worldwide. Oxford is a registered trade mark of
Oxford University Press in the UK and in certain other countries

Published in the United States of America by Oxford University Press
198 Madison Avenue, New York, NY 10016, United States of America

British Library Cataloguing in Publication Data
Data available

Library of Congress Control Number: 2015938212

ISBN 978–0–19–871911–3

Printed in Great Britain by Clays Ltd, St Ives plc

Oxford University Press makes no representation, express or implied, that the
drug dosages in this book are correct. Readers must therefore always check
the product information and clinical procedures with the most up-to-date
published product information and data sheets provided by the manufacturers
and the most recent codes of conduct and safety regulations. The authors and
the publishers do not accept responsibility or legal liability for any errors in the
text or for the misuse or misapplication of material in this work. Except where
otherwise stated, drug dosages and recommendations are for the non-pregnant
adult who is not breast-feeding

Links to third party websites are provided by Oxford in good faith and
for information only. Oxford disclaims any responsibility for the materials
contained in any third party website referenced in this work.

Contents

Abbreviations

ANP	atrial natriuretic peptide
ANV	actual number of nightly voids
5-ARI	5-alpha reductase inhibitor
AUA	American Urological Association
AUA-SI	American Urological Association symptom index
AVP	arginine vasopressin
BOO	bladder outlet obstruction
BPE	benign prostatic enlargement
BPH	benign prostatic hyperplasia
BPO	benign prostatic obstruction
CI	confidence interval
CT	computed tomography
EEG	electroencephalogram
ER	extended release
FDA	Food and Drug Administration
FVC	frequency/volume chart
GFR	glomerular filtration rate
HADS	hospital anxiety and depression scale
HIFU	high-intensity focused ultrasound
HUS	hours of uninterrupted sleep
ICIQ	International Consultation on Incontinence Questionnaire
ICS	International Continence Society
IPSS	International Prostate Symptom Score
LUTS	lower urinary tract symptoms
mOsmol	milliosmole
MRI	magnetic resonance imaging
NBCi	nocturnal bladder capacity index
Ni	nocturia index
NPI	nocturnal polyuria index
N-QoL	Nocturia Quality of Life
NSAID	non-steroidal anti-inflammatory drug
OAB	overactive bladder
OCAS	oral controlled absorption system
OR	odds ratio

PDE5i	phosphodiesterase-5 inhibitor
PNV	predicted number of nightly voids
PSA	prostate-specific antigen
PSQI	Pittsburgh Sleep Quality Index
PTNS	percutaneous posterior tibial nerve stimulation
PVR	post-void residual
Qmax	maximum urinary flow rate
QoL	quality of life
RCT	randomized controlled trial
SD	standard deviation
SNS	sacral nerve stimulation
TUIP	transurethral incision of the prostate
TUMT	transurethral microwave therapy
TUNA	transurethral needle ablation
TURP	transurethral resection of the prostate
TUVP	transurethral electrosurgical vaporization of the prostate
UWIN	Urgency, Weak stream, Incomplete emptying, and Nocturia
VLAP	visual laser ablation of the prostate
WMD	weighted mean difference

Contributors

Editors

Paul Abrams

Professor of Urology
Bristol Urological Institute
Southmead Hospital
Bristol, UK

Hashim Hashim

Consultant Urological Surgeon and
Director of the Urodynamics Unit
Bristol Urological Institute
Southmead Hospital
Bristol, UK

Contributors

Roger Dmochowski

Department of Urology
Vanderbilt University School of Medicine
Nashville, TN, USA

Marcus Drake

Senior Lecturer in Urology
School of Clinical Sciences
University of Bristol
Bristol, UK

Haerin Lee

Department of Urology
Vanderbilt University School of Medicine
Nashville, TN, USA

David James Osborn

Department of Urology
Vanderbilt University School of Medicine
Nashville, TN, USA

Dudley Robinson

Consultant Urogynaecologist/Honorary
Senior Lecturer
Department of Urogynaecology
King's College Hospital
London, UK

Daniel P. Verges

Chief Resident
Department of Urology
SUNY Downstate College of Medicine
Brooklyn, NY, USA

Jeffrey P. Weiss

Professor and Chair
Department of Urology
SUNY Downstate College of Medicine
Brooklyn, NY, USA

Chapter 1

Definitions used in lower urinary tract symptoms

Hashim Hashim

Key points

- Nocturia is defined as the complaint that the individual has to wake at night one or more times to void. It has to be preceded and followed by sleep.
- It is part of storage lower urinary tract symptoms.
- It is important to differentiate nocturia from nocturnal enuresis which is wetting the bed at night whilst asleep.
- The definition of nocturia does not take into account the degree of bother or the aetiology.

1.1 Definitions

Lower urinary tract symptoms (LUTS) can be divided into storage, voiding, and post-micturition symptoms [1]. Storage symptoms occur when the bladder is filling with urine; voiding symptoms occur when the individual is voiding, and post-micturition symptoms occur after the person has finished voiding (Table 1.1).

Nocturia is part of the storage symptoms and, in 2002, has been defined by International Continence Society (ICS) as the complaint that an individual has to wake at night one or more times to void. Prior to 2002, there was no official definition. In 2010, the ICS definition of nocturia has been slightly modified to the complaint of interruption of sleep one or more times because of the need to micturate. Each void is preceded and followed by sleep [2].

It is important to note that aetiology and bother are not part of the definition of nocturia. In other words, the definition does not include the cause of the nocturia. If a person wakes up every night because they have a partner who snores, or because they have noisy neighbours or a child who is crying, and they decide to pass urine during the night when they wake up, then, by definition, this is nocturia. It is, however, non-pathological nocturia, i.e. the definition does not take into account whether there is pathology or not. Even if pathology is included, nocturia has multifactorial aetiology, as will be seen in Chapter 2, and it would be difficult to include a definition for every pathology.

The current definition also does not include the degree of bother and impact on quality of life (QoL). Studies have shown that nocturia does not become bothersome until the individual gets up two or more times to void at night [3]. However, what the current definition aims to do is to standardize the usage of the term, and any extra information will have to be included in any form of communication that may account for the aetiology and degree of bother of nocturia.

Table 1.1 Definitions of lower urinary tract symptoms standardized by the International Continence Society	
Storage LUTS	
Nocturia	The complaint that the individual has to wake at night one or more times to void
Increased daytime frequency	The complaint by the patient who considers that he/she voids too often by day
Urgency	The complaint of a sudden compelling desire to pass urine which is difficult to defer
Urinary incontinence	The complaint of any involuntary leakage of urine
Voiding LUTS	
Slow stream	Reported by the individual as his or her perception of reduced urine flow, usually compared to previous performance or in comparison to others
Intermittent stream (intermittency)	The term used when the individual describes urine flow which stops and starts, on one or more occasions, during micturition
Hesitancy	The term used when an individual describes difficulty in initiating micturition, resulting in a delay in the onset of voiding, after the individual is ready to pass urine
Straining to void	Describes the muscular effort used to either initiate, maintain, or improve the urinary stream. Suprapubic pressure may be used to initiate or maintain flow
Terminal dribble	The term used when an individual describes a prolonged final part of micturition, when the flow has slowed to a trickle/dribble
Post-micturition LUTS	
Feeling of incomplete emptying	A self-explanatory term for a feeling experienced by the individual after passing urine
Post-micturition dribble	The term used when an individual describes the involuntary loss of urine immediately after he or she has finished passing urine, usually after leaving the toilet in men or after rising from the toilet in women

Adapted from *Neurourology and Urodynamics*, 21(2), Abrams *et al.*, 'The standardisation of terminology of lower urinary tract function: Report from the standardisation sub-committee of the International, pp. 167–178, Copyright (2002), with permission from John Wiley and Sons.

1.2 **Criteria for definition of nocturia**

There are certain agreed criteria that need to be fulfilled before an individual is labelled as having nocturia. These include:

1. each void must be preceded and followed by sleep, i.e. the first morning void is not included when the number of episodes of nocturia is being counted (see example in Chapter 3)

2. it is independent of the trigger for waking

3. it depends on the time spent sleeping, and not on the time spent in bed, i.e. it does NOT include:

   i. voids after going to bed, but before going to sleep

   ii. voids that prevent from going back to sleep.

These criteria can be slightly confusing if a person goes to bed at 10 p.m. and reads a book, then passes urine at 10.30 p.m. and goes back to bed, and then falls asleep at 11 p.m.! This is part of night-time frequency, but NOT nocturia, because it has to be preceded and followed by sleep to be nocturia. If, however, after falling asleep at 11 p.m., the person wakes up at 3 a.m. and then goes back to bed to sleep, then this would be considered nocturia (see example in Chapter 3).

1.3 Terms related to nocturia

Nocturia and the associated terms (Table 1.2) are mainly derived from the bladder diary. It is important to note that it is not possible to treat patients who complain of nocturia without the use of a bladder diary, ideally over a 3-day period, e.g. ICIQ-Bladder Diary (see Chapter 3).

Table 1.2 Terms related to nocturia	
Term	Definition
Nocturnal urine volume	Total volume of urine passed during the night, including the first morning void. This is an important definition that can also be confusing! When calculating nocturia episodes, the first morning void is not included, because it is not followed by sleep. However, when calculating nocturnal volume, the volume voided from the first morning void needs to be included, as it is urine being stored in the bladder during the night
	A nocturnal urine production of >6.4 mL/kg per sleep cycle is suggestive of nocturnal polyuria [4]
Rate of nocturnal urine production	Nocturnal urine volume/time asleep (i.e. night); measured in mL/min
	More than 0.9 mL/min is suggestive of nocturnal polyuria (about 450 mL per 8 h of sleep)
Nocturnal polyuria	Nocturnal urine volume >20–33% of total 24-hour urine volume (age-dependent): • 33% in elderly, e.g. >65 • >20% in younger individuals • 20–33% in 'middle age'
Nocturnal polyuria index (NPI)	Nocturnal urine volume/24-hour voided volume
24-hour voided volume	Total volume of urine voided during a 24-hour period (1st void to be discarded; 24 hours begin at the time of the next void)
24-hour global polyuria	24-hour voided volume in excess of 2800 mL (in 70 kg person, i.e. >40 mL/kg)
Night	The period of time between going to bed with the intention of sleeping and waking with the intention of arising
Night-time frequency	The number of voids recorded from the time the individual goes to bed with the intention of going to sleep to the time the individual wakes with the intention of rising. It relates to the total time in bed. Therefore, it is the number of voids recorded from the time of going to bed to the time of rising and includes: • voids after going to bed, but before going to sleep • nocturia episodes • voids in the early morning, but the individual goes back to bed but not to sleep • depends on the time in bed

3

(continued)

Table 1.2 Continued	
Term	Definition
First morning void	The first void after waking with the intention of rising
Maximum voided volume	The largest single voided volume measured in a 24-hour period
Nocturnal enuresis	Voiding or wetting the bed whilst asleep, i.e. the individual is unaware and is in a state of sleep and is not awake. In other words, it is urinary incontinence whilst asleep
Nocturia index (Ni)	Nocturnal urine volume/maximum voided volume [5] >1: nocturia occurs because maximum voided volume is smaller than nocturnal urine volume >1.5: nocturia secondary to nocturnal urine overproduction in excess of maximum bladder capacity, i.e. nocturnal polyuria
Nocturnal bladder capacity index (NBCi)	Actual number of nightly voids (ANV) minus predicted number of nightly voids (PNV) (PNV = Ni − 1) [6] >0: nocturia occurring at volumes less than maximum voided volume >1.3: reduced bladder capacity as a cause of nocturia. The higher the value, the more likely it is the nocturia is due to reduced bladder capacity

1.4 Conclusion

In 2002, ICS defined nocturia as the complaint that an individual has to wake up one or more times to void. This definition means that the person must be awake before each void and goes back to sleep after voiding.

The aim of the ICS definition was to standardize the nomenclature. Obviously, this definition is not without its limitations, the main one being that it does not differentiate between pathological and non-pathological causes of nocturia. Also it does not apply to shift workers who often have disrupted and poor sleep as their natural circadian rhythm is altered. Furthermore, individuals whose sleep is disturbed by their bladder, so that they go to the toilet but cannot get back to sleep again, are not included, even if that voiding episode leaves them tired.

Previous definitions, such as having at least two voids or three voids at night, attempt to encompass bothersomeness without specifically asking the patient 'How much bother does getting up at night cause you?'.

Therefore, with this in mind, ICS suggested that nocturia is a 'condition', and not a 'disease', since a condition is defined as 'a state of being, specifically in reference to physical and mental health or well-being'. A disease, on the other hand, is a condition of abnormal vital function involving any structure, part, or system. The understanding of the distinctions between the different terminologies is very important, and it is equally vital that all health care providers are speaking the same 'language' when it comes to nocturia, as this has implications when patients report 'nocturia' and therefore on clinical trial results and on the treatment of patients. This distinction has to be clearly explained to patients when filling out frequency/volume charts as well.

References

1. Abrams P, *et al*. The standardisation of terminology of lower urinary tract function: report from the Standardisation Sub-committee of the International Continence Society. *Neurourol Urodyn*. 2002;**21**:167–78.

2. Toozs-Hobson P, *et al*. An International Urogynecological Association (IUGA)/International Continence Society (ICS) joint report on the terminology for reporting outcomes of surgical procedures for pelvic organ prolapse. *Neurourol Urodyn*. 2012;**31**:415–21.

3. Tikkinen KA, *et al*. Nocturia frequency, bother, and quality of life: how often is too often? A population-based study in Finland. *Eur Urol*. 2010;**57**:488–96.

4. Matthiesen TB, *et al*. Nocturnal polyuria and natriuresis in male patients with nocturia and lower urinary tract symptoms. *J Urol*. 1996;**156**:1292–9.

5. Weiss JP, *et al*. Nocturia in adults: etiology and classification. *Neurourol Urodyn*. 1998;**17**:467–72.

6. Burton C, *et al*. Reference values for the Nocturnal Bladder Capacity Index. *Neurourol Urodyn*. 2011;**30**:52–7.

Chapter 2

Nocturia: epidemiology and pathophysiology

Dudley Robinson

Key points
• Nocturia is the most prevalent lower urinary tract symptom.
• The prevalence of nocturia increases with age.
• Nocturia significantly affects quality of life.
• Nocturia has several risk factors, including age and obesity.
• Nocturia has multifactorial aetiology, including urological and non-urological causes:
• urological causes include abnormal bladder function
• non-urological causes include medical conditions causing, for example, excessive urine production and/or social conditions that can cause sleep disturbances.

2.1 Introduction

Nocturia, defined as the complaint that the individual has to wake at night one or more times to void [1], is a bothersome condition that is known to have a considerable impact on QoL. The symptom of nocturia is known to lead to sleep disturbance which adversely affects daytime functioning and may also lead to impaired physical and mental performance. As a consequence, nocturia may have implications regarding daytime productivity and long-term mental health.

In addition, nocturia forms part of the symptom complex of overactive bladder (OAB)—defined as urinary urgency, usually accompanied by frequency and nocturia, with or without urgency urinary incontinence, in the absence of urinary tract infection or other obvious pathology [2].

This chapter aims to review the epidemiology and aetiology of patients with nocturia, as well as give an overview of the pathophysiology.

2.2 Epidemiology

2.2.1 Prevalence

The prevalence of nocturia is known to increase with age. Whilst 4% of children have been reported to experience nocturia [3], this rises to 59% in women and 67% in men aged 50–59 years, and in 72% of women and 91% of men over the age of 80 years [4]. This is supported by a questionnaire-based survey of community-dwelling women, in which the prevalence of nocturia (defined as two or more voids) increased with age from 9% in women below the age of 20 years to 51% in those older than 80 years of age [5].

More recently, the prevalence of nocturia has been reported in the FINNO study [6]. This was a large Finnish questionnaire-based case-control study of 6000 subjects, aged 18–79 years, performed in 2003–2004. Overall, one in eight men and women reported at least two voids per night, and one-third reported one void per night. The prevalence of nocturia was greater in younger women, as compared to younger men, although this became similar in the 6th and 7th decades. In the older age groups, however, men were found to have a higher prevalence when compared to women.

These findings are supported by the Krimpen study conducted amongst 1688 elderly men aged 50–78 years in the Netherlands. Nocturia was assessed using frequency–volume charts, and overall 1.5 voids per night or more were present in 60% of men aged 70–78 years, whilst 20% reported 2.5 voids or more [7].

2.2.2 Incidence

Whilst there are many studies reporting the prevalence of nocturia, there are far fewer studies investigating the incidence, perhaps reflecting the difficulty in performing longitudinal studies.

A community-based study amongst adults over the age of 60 years has been reported in North America [8]. Of the 738 subjects with no symptoms of nocturia, 34.6% reported nocturia (≥2 voids) at follow-up, giving an incidence of 213/1000 person years. Of the 357 subjects who had ≥2 nocturnal voids at baseline, 66.3% reported one or fewer episodes at follow-up, giving a remission rate of 497/1000 patient years.

Although there is a paucity of longitudinal studies reported in women, there are some data investigating long-term incidence in men. In the Krimpen study, the overall incidence and remission rates of nocturia (≥2 voids) were 23.9% and 36.7%, respectively, after 2.1 years. In general, the incidence was found to be highest amongst the more elderly, and lower amongst the younger subjects, and the prevalence rate increased over time [7].

A questionnaire-based study has also been reported in Finland, investigating the incidence of nocturia in men over a 10-year period [9]. Overall, the crude incidence for one nocturnal void was 75 new cases per 1000 person years during the first 5 years, and 126 new cases per 1000 person years during the next 5 years.

In summary, the available evidence from longitudinal studies would appear to suggest that, whilst nocturia increases with age, it also has a fluctuating course, and, in some cases, remission may occur.

2.2.3 Overactive bladder

The symptom of nocturia is also included in the symptom complex of OAB. Prevalence data from a large North American study of 5204 adults have indicated that 16.9% of women complain of symptoms of OAB [10], and this is confirmed by the results of a European population-based study of 16 776 men and women which found the overall prevalence to be 16.6% in individuals over the age of 40 years [11]. Whilst 60% had sought a medical consultation regarding their LUTS, only 27% were currently receiving treatment. More recently, a further population-based survey of LUTS in Canada, Germany, Italy, Sweden, and the United Kingdom has reported on 19 165 men and women over the age of 18 years [12]. Overall, 11.8% were found to complain of symptoms suggestive of OAB, and 64.3% reported at least one urinary symptom. Nocturia was the most prevalent LUTS, being reported by 48.6% of men and 54.5% of women.

These findings are also supported by a large population-based Canadian study of 1000 men and women. Over 50% of respondents reported one or more LUTS, with nocturia being the most commonly reported in 36% of subjects. Overall, the prevalence was found to increase with age, and the median duration of symptoms was 5 years [13].

Consequently, whilst nocturia may be an isolated symptom, it may also be associated with a number of other LUTS and may often be the most commonly reported symptom associated with OAB.

2.3 Risk factors

2.3.1 Age

The prevalence of nocturia is known to increase with age in both men and women, and the incidence is also known to increase with ageing. A community-based study from North America has shown that, whilst <5% of 18–24 year olds reported two voids per night, this increased to approximately 15% and 25% of 45–54 year olds and 65–74 year olds, respectively [14]. In addition, childhood nocturia has also been shown to predict nocturia in later life [15].

2.3.2 Gender

Although there are no major differences in the prevalence of nocturia in men and women, some studies have found a higher prevalence in younger women, when compared to young men, although this difference is lost by middle age [16].

2.3.3 Obesity

Obesity has been shown to be associated with a threefold risk of nocturia in middle-aged women [17] and a twofold risk in men. This has also been confirmed in the Tampere Aging Male Urologic Study (TAMUS) which demonstrated that obese men over 50 years old had double the risk of nocturia [18].

2.3.4 Lifestyle factors

In general, there would appear to be no association between nocturia and alcohol [19] or caffeine consumption [18]. In addition, there is no association of nocturia with smoking [19].

Overall, physical exercise would appear to be protective against LUTS in men [20] and nocturia in women [21], and exercise has been shown to improve the symptoms of nocturia in a non-randomized trial [22].

2.3.5 Ethnicity

Evidence from North American studies has shown that African Americans are twice as likely to report symptoms of nocturia as other ethnic groups [23], and care-seeking black women have also been shown to report nocturia more commonly [24]. A further small study in Scotland has demonstrated that nocturia is commoner in Caucasian men, compared to Asian men [25].

2.3.6 Pregnancy and childbirth

Nocturia is a commonly reported symptom in pregnancy and has been shown to increase during gestation [26]. In addition, parous women have been shown to report more nocturia than nulliparous women, although there is no difference between primiparous and multiparous women, suggesting that the effect is due to pregnancy itself, rather than deliver [27]. In addition, there is no difference in incidence, following vaginal delivery and Caesarean section [28].

2.3.7 Menopause

The risk of nocturia has been shown to increase, following the menopause, and Danish [29] and Finnish [27] population-based studies have reported more than double the risk. Whilst the evidence regarding the risk of nocturia associated with systemic hormone therapy is contradictory [30, 31], there is no increased risk with vaginal oestrogens [32].

2.3.8 Others

Nocturia has also been found to be associated with metabolic syndrome, hypertension, winter season, increased C-reactive protein levels, lower educational attainment, low testosterone levels in men, and/or low vitamin D levels, without very clear explanation to date. No clear genetic predisposition has yet been found, although twin studies point toward a possible genetic risk in women.

2.4 Aetiology

The causes of nocturia are often multifactorial and may be associated with a number of different medical and social conditions (Box 2.1). In clinical practice, however, nocturia is usually associated with an increase in nocturnal urine production, problems related to bladder storage, and sleep pattern abnormalities.

Patients with nocturia can be categorized into four broad types, according to bladder function and urine production:

1. abnormal bladder function + normal urine production
2. abnormal bladder function + excessive urine production
3. normal bladder function + normal urine production
4. normal bladder function + excessive urine production.

2.4.1 24-hour polyuria

Polyuria is a condition characterized by the excretion of an excessively large volume of urine over a 24-hour period, day and night, usually with a normal night/day ratio (~0.25), and is defined as a urine output in excess of 40 mL/kg body weight [1]. Physiologically, the rate of urine production is controlled by two factors: the concentration of urine and the rate of solute excretion. The former is determined by the antidiuretic hormone arginine vasopressin (AVP), which acts upon the distal tubules and collecting ducts within the kidney tubule to increase the amount of water reabsorbed from the glomerular filtrate. The latter is composed mostly of urea, sodium, and potassium, and the rate of excretion is determined by diet and other factors influencing protein metabolism and the extracellular fluid volume (Box 2.2).

AVP is a peptide hormone that increases water permeability of the kidney's collecting duct and distal convoluted tubule by inducing the translocation of aquaporin-CD water channels in the plasma membrane of the collecting duct of the kidney nephron. It also increases peripheral vascular resistance, which, in turn, increases arterial blood pressure. It plays a key role in homeostasis by the regulation of water, glucose, and salts in the blood. It is derived from a

---

Box 2.1 Conditions associated with the symptom of nocturia

Ageing
Psychogenic
Behavioural
Sleep disturbance
Polyuria
Bladder storage problems
Neurological disease

Box 2.2 Causes of 24-hour polyuria

Diabetes mellitus
Insulin-dependent diabetes (type I)
Non-insulin-dependent diabetes (type II)

Diabetes insipidus
Pituitary (central)—deficiency in AVP at the pituitary level
Nephrogenic—renal insensitivity to AVP
Gestational—related to pregnancy

Primary polydipsia
Psychogenic—related to psychological and/or cognitive impairment
Dipsogenic—caused by a primary abnormality in the thirst mechanism
Iatrogenic—caused by self-induced water intoxication

Drugs
Diuretics, selective serotonin reuptake inhibitors, calcium channel blockers, tetracycline, lithium, carbonic anhydrase inhibitors

Hypercalcaemia

---

pre-prohormone precursor that is synthesized in the hypothalamus and stored in vesicles in the posterior pituitary.

2.4.2 **Nocturnal polyuria**

Nocturnal polyuria refers specifically to the production of an abnormally high volume of urine during sleep. Clearly, whilst many of the causes of polyuria may also cause nocturnal polyuria, there are other conditions which may present with the symptom of nocturia. These may be summarized as those that cause a water diuresis alone and those that cause a combined solute and water diuresis (Box 2.3).

Water diuresis (urine osmolarity <300 mOsmol/L; specific gravity <1.010) is caused by a low basal serum vasopressin level, resulting in a high urinary volume. Solute diuresis (urine

---

Box 2.3 Causes of nocturnal polyuria

Water diuresis
Circadian defect in secretion or action of AVP (including central nervous system lesions of the hypothalamic–pituitary axis, Parkinson's disease, multiple sclerosis)

Primary—idiopathic

Secondary—excessive evening intake of fluid

Solute/water diuresis
Peripheral oedema/atrial natriuretic factor (ANF) secretion: congestive heart failure, autonomic neuropathy, venous stasis, lymphostasis, hepatic failure, hypoalbuminaemia/malnutrition, nephrotic syndrome

Autonomic nervous system dysfunction

Sleep apnoea syndrome

Renal failure/renal tubular dysfunction (including diabetes mellitus and albuminuria)
Oestrogen deficiency

Drugs: diuretics, ethanol, steroids

---

osmolarity ≥300 mOsmol/L; specific gravity ≥1.010) is the result of increased delivery to the collecting tubule of any solute, such as glucose, sodium, and chloride, urea, mannitol, or radiocontrast.

In nocturnal polyuria, there is a high urine output at night only, with an abnormal night/day ratio (>0.25). A more accurate way of calculating whether a patient has nocturnal polyuria is using the NPI. If the patient is 65 years or older and the NPI is >33%, then the patient has nocturnal polyuria. If the patient is younger than 35 years, then nocturnal polyuria is defined as an NPI > 20%. Between the ages of 35 and 65, the value of the NPI is somewhere between 20% and 33%, and probably about 25%.

$$NPI = [Night\text{-}time\ urine\ volume\ (mL) / Total\ 24\text{-}hour\ urine\ volume\ (mL)] \times 100$$

2.4.3 Bladder storage problems

In addition to causes secondary to urine overproduction, men and women may present with nocturia secondary to bladder storage problems and lower urinary tract dysfunction (Box 2.4). A reduced functional capacity secondary to detrusor overactivity or extrinsic bladder compression may lead to symptoms of nocturia, as may chronic voiding problems. In addition, nocturia is a symptom suggestive of OAB and may be associated with diurnal frequency, urgency, and urgency incontinence.

2.4.4 Sleep disturbance

Sleep disturbance may be a cause or consequence of nocturia, and it is important to elicit, when taking a history, whether the patient wakes to void or simply empties their bladder, whilst awake, for another reason. Sleep disorders causing nocturia may be related to concomitant medical or psychiatric conditions (Box 2.5).

Box 2.4 Causes of nocturia secondary to bladder storage problems

Reduced functional bladder capacity
Extrinsic compression (uterine fibroids, urogenital prolapse, ovarian tumour)

Bladder pain syndrome
Interstitial cystitis, chronic cystitis

Detrusor overactivity
Idiopathic
Neurogenic (Parkinson's disease, multiple sclerosis, spinal cord injury, stroke)

Overactive bladder (OAB), bladder outlet obstruction (BOO)
Voiding problems and post-void residual (PVR) urine
BOO, including benign prostatic obstruction (BPO), urethral stricture, uterine fibroids and urogenital prolapse, and detrusor underactivity

Urogenital ageing
Urogenital atrophy due to oestrogen deficiency

Lower urinary tract cancer

Bladder ageing

Lower urinary tract calculi

Box 2.5 Causes of nocturia related to sleep disturbance

Sleep disorders
Insomnia
Sleep apnoea
Periodic leg movements
Narcolepsy
Arousal disorders: sleepwalking, nightmares

Medical disorders
Cardiac failure
Chronic obstructive pulmonary disease
Endocrine disorders: thyrotoxicosis, acromegaly

Neurological conditions
Parkinson's disease
Dementia
Epilepsy

Psychiatric conditions
Depression
Anxiety

Chronic pain disorders
Rheumatoid arthritis
Osteoarthritis

Alcohol/drugs
Consumption and withdrawal

Medication
Corticosteroids, diuretics, beta-adrenergic antagonists, thyroid hormones, psychotropics, anti-epileptics

2.4.4.1 *Nocturia and sleep*

Sleep is an essential, recurrent physiological state of unconsciousness and inactivity of the voluntary muscles that follows a characteristic circadian rhythm in all biological individuals, including humans [33]. Whilst the true need for sleep remains poorly understood, sleep is known to be essential in order to maintain physical and mental functioning. Sleep deprivation is associated with daytime sleepiness, lack of concentration and coordination, reduction in creativity, and alteration of mood [34].

Nocturia is known to be an important cause of sleep disturbance, and, in a Dutch cross-sectional epidemiological study, nocturia and worries were found to be the most important cause of sleep disturbance in adults over 50 years old [4]. The effects of nocturia on sleep disturbance have also been investigated amongst an elderly population in Sweden. Nocturia was found to be associated with an increased prevalence of sleep disorders, poorer quality of sleep, and increased daytime fatigue [35]. More recently, there is some evidence to suggest that the integrity of the immune system is affected by sleep deprivation [36] and that sleep is important in maintaining host defences [37]. Overall, there is some evidence to suggest that sleep disturbance is associated with increased mortality [38].

Sleep apnoea has also been associated with nocturia. The precise relationship between sleep apnoea and nocturia has not been thoroughly studied, but it seems to be related to increased pressure in the right side of the heart. Obstructive sleep apnoea is caused by a blockage of the upper airway when the soft tissue in the rear of the throat collapses and closes during sleep. This sets off a series of physiological processes—oxygen supply decreases; carbon dioxide levels increase, and the blood becomes more acidic, resulting in bradycardia and pulmonary vasoconstriction. The patient then wakes up to breathe, by which time the heart rate increases and the heart senses a false signal of fluid overload which results in the secretion of atrial natriuretic peptide (ANP) to get rid of sodium and water, resulting in nocturia. The worse the sleep apnoea, the worse the nocturia. Treatment of sleep apnoea with continuous positive airway pressure is usually a very successful way of reducing nocturia in these patients.

2.5 Economic impact of nocturia

The effect of nocturia and subsequent sleep deprivation has also been investigated, in terms of productivity and utility, in a study of 203 subjects and 80 controls in Sweden [39]. Overall, the study group with nocturia were found to have a significantly lower level of vitality and utility, when compared to the control group, and were also found to have a greater impairment of work and activity. In general, women were more affected than men. The authors concluded that nocturia was associated with a significant impairment of daytime functioning, and this may lead to a significant level of indirect and intangible costs.

2.6 Conclusions

Nocturia is a common LUTS which is known to adversely affect QoL and lead to sleep deprivation and a reduction in daytime productivity. Whilst some patients may present with nocturia as an isolated symptom, many may complain of nocturia as part of the symptoms of OAB in association with urgency, urgency incontinence, and daytime frequency.

The evidence would suggest that the prevalence and incidence of nocturia increase with age, and risk factors associated with developing symptoms include ethnicity, obesity, and menopausal status. In addition, many medical conditions may be associated with nocturia, including diabetes mellitus, hypertension, and coronary disease.

Whilst the pathophysiology of nocturia is often multifactorial, the commonest causes include 24-hour polyuria, nocturnal polyuria, reduced bladder storage, and sleep disturbance. Consequently, the management of patients complaining of symptoms of nocturia should focus on investigating and treating each underlying cause, in addition to effectively managing the patient's symptoms.

References

1. Van Kerrebroeck P, et al. The standardisation of terminology of nocturia: report from the Standardisation Subcommittee of the International Continence Society. Neurourol Urodynam. 2002;21:179–83.

2. Haylen BT, et al. An International Urogynaecological Association (IUGA)/International Continence Society (ICS) joint report on the terminology for female pelvic floor dysfunction. Int Urogynecol J. 2010;21:5–26.

3. Mattsson S. Urinary incontinence and nocturia in healthy school children. Acta Paediatr. 1994;83:950–4.

4. Middlekoop HA, et al. Subjective sleep characteristics of 1485 males and females aged 50–93: effects of sex and age, and factors related to self-evaluated quality of sleep. J Gerontol Biol Sci Med Sci. 1996;51:108–15.

5. Swithinbank LV, et al . Female urinary symptoms: age prevalence in a community dwelling population using a validated questionnaire. Neurourol Urodyn. 1998;16:432–4.

6. Tikkinen KA, et al. Is nocturia equally commen amonst men and women? A population based study in Finland. J Urol. 2006;175:596–600.

7. Blanker MH, *et al*. Normal voiding patterns and determinants of increased diurnal and nocturnal voiding frequency in elderly men. *J Urol*. 2000;**164**:1201–5.

8. Herzog AR and Fultz NH. Prevalence and incidence of urinary incontinence in community dwelling populations. *J Am Geriatr Soc*. 1990;**38**:273–81.

9. Hakkinen JT, *et al*. Incidence of nocturia in 50–80 year old Finnish men. *J Urol*. 2006;**176**:2541–5.

10. Stewart WF, *et al*. Prevalence and burden of overactive bladder in the United States. *World J Urol*. 2003;**20**:327–36.

11. Milsom I, *et al*. How widespread are the symptoms of an overactive bladder and how are they managed? A population based prevalence study. *BJU Int*. 2001;**87**:760–6.

12. Irwin DE, *et al*. Population-based survey of urinary incontinence, overactive bladder and other lower urinary tract symptoms in five countries: results of the EPIC study. *Eur Urol*. 2006;**50**:1306–14.

13. Herschorn S, *et al*. A population based study of urinary symptoms and incontinence: the Canadian Urinary Bladder Survey. *BJU Int*. 2008;**101**:52–8.

14. Coyne KS, *et al*. The prevalence of nocturia and its effect on health related quality of life and sleep in a community sample in the USA. *BJU Int*. 2003;**92**:948–54.

15. Fitzgerald MP, *et al*. Childhood urinary symptoms predict adult overactive bladder symptoms. *J Urol*. 2006;**175**:989–93.

16. Hunskaar S. Epidemiology of nocturia. *BJU Int*. 2005;**96** Suppl 1:4–7.

17. Coyne KS, *et al*. Racial differences in the prevalence of overactive bladder in the United States from the Epidemiology of LUTS (EpiLUTS) Study. *Urology*. 2012;**79**:95–101.

18. Shiri R, *et al*. The effects of lifestyle factors on the incidence of nocturia. *J Urol*. 2008;**180**:2059–62.

19. Tikkinen KA, *et al*. A systematic evaluation of factors associated with nocturia—the population based FINNO study. *Am J Epidemiol*. 2009;**170**:361–8.

20. Rohrmann S, *et al*. Association of cigarette smoking, alcohol consumption and physical activity with lower urinary tract symptoms in older American men: findings from the third national Health and Nutrition Examination Survey. *BJU Int*. 2005;**96**:77–82.

21. Asplund R and Aberg HE. Nocturia in relation to body mass index, smoking and some other lifestyle factors in women. *Climacteric*. 2004;**7**:267–73.

22. Soda T, *et al*. Efficacy of non-drug lifestyle measures for the treatment of nocturia. *J Urol*. 2010;**184**:1000–4.

23. Fitzgerald MP, *et al*., BACH survey investigators. The association of nocturia with cardiac disease, diabetes, body mass index age and diuretic use. *J Urol*. 2007;**177**:1385–9.

24. Sze EH, *et al*. Prevalence of urinary incontinence symptoms among black, white and Hispanic women. *Obstet Gynaecol*. 2002;**99**:572–5.

25. Mariappan P, *et al*. Nocturia, nocturia indices and variables from frequency volume charts are significantly different in Asian and Caucasian men with lower urinary tract symptoms: a prospective comparison study. *BJU Int*. 2007;**100**:332–6.

26. Sharma JB, *et al*. Prevalence of urinary incontinence and other urological problems during pregnancy: a questionnaire based study. *Arch Gynecol Obstet*. 2009;**279**:845–51.

27. Tikkinen KA, *et al*. Reproductive factors associated with nocturia and urinary urgency in women: a population based study in Finland. *Am J Obstet Gynecol*. 2008;**199**:153.e1–12.

28. Ekstrom A, *et al*. Planned Caesarean section versus planned vaginal delivery: comparison of lower urinary tract symptoms. *Int Urogynaecol J Pelvic Floor Dysfunct*. 2007;**18**:133–9.

29. Alling Moller L, Lose G, and Jorgensen T. Risk factors for lower urinary tract symptoms in women 40 to 60 years of age. *Obstet Gynaecol*. 2000;**96**:446–51.

30. Asplund R and Aberg HE. Development of nocturia in relation to health, age and the menopause. *Maturitas*. 2005;**51**:358–62.

31. Cardozo L, *et al*. Oestriol in the treatment of postmenopausal urgency: a multicentre study. *Maturitas*. 1993;**18**:47–53.

32. Liapis A, *et al*. The use of oestradiol therapy in postmenopausal women after TVTO anti-incontinence surgery. *Maturitas*. 2010;**66**:101–6.

33. Tobler I. Why do we sleep? Contributions from animal research. *Ther Umsch*. 2000;**57**:417–20.

34. Bromen JE, Lundh LG, and Hetta J. Insufficient sleep in the general population. *Neurophysiol Clin.* 1996;**26**:30–9.

35. Asplund R and Aberg H. Health of the elderly with regard to sleep and nocturnal micturition. *Scand J Prim Health Care.* 1992;**10**:98–104.

36. Benca RM and Quintas J. Sleep and host defences: a review. *Sleep.* 1997;**20**:1027–37.

37. Irwin M, *et al.* Partial night sleep deprivation reduces natural killer and cellular immune responses in humans. *FASEB J.* 1996;**10**:643–53.

38. Mattiasson I, *et al.* Threat of unemployment and cardiovascular risk factors: longitudinal study of quality of life of sleep and serum cholesterol concentrations in men threatened with redundancy. *BMJ.* 1990;**301**:461–6.

39. Kobelt G, Borgstrom F, and Mattiasson A. Productivity, vitality and utility in a group of healthy professionally active individuals with nocturia. *BJU Int.* 2003;**91**:190–5.

Chapter 3

Assessment of nocturia

Marcus Drake

Key points

- Patients suffering from nocturia need a thorough medical and surgical history and focused clinical examination.
- Baseline investigations required for patients suffering with nocturia include:
  - height and weight to calculate body mass index
  - bladder diary, e.g. the ICIQ-Bladder Diary
  - symptom and quality of life questionnaires, e.g. ICIQ-N and ICIQ-NQoL
  - urinalysis, e.g. 'dipstick'
  - flow rate and post-void residual measurement
  - biochemical tests, e.g. renal electrolytes.
- Further urological investigations, such as urodynamics, cystoscopy, or imaging, are not indicated, unless an abnormality is suspected on baseline investigations and after failure of conservative and medical therapy.
- Patients are usually referred to the urologist for nocturia. However, following a thorough investigation, patients may need to be referred to another specialty to exclude potential systemic diagnoses, such as sleep disorders, sleep apnoea, or endocrine dysfunction.

3.1 Introduction

Clinical assessment of nocturia aims to establish the severity and QoL impact of the symptom, and also to try to understand underlying mechanisms in individuals affected. In general, more severe nocturia is likely to reflect a worse underlying problem, and it may well have a greater impact on QoL. However, bother levels do not necessarily correspond with symptom severity, since individual attitudes may differ. Sometimes younger people report bother from the symptom, whilst older people might be more accepting of nocturia of similar severity. Accordingly, severity and bother should both be considered.

Nocturia is not only a LUTS, but also an aspect of homeostatic control. Urine output is determined physiologically to eliminate excess free water (diuresis) or excess salt (natriuresis); some conditions can lead to excessive free water or salt excretion beyond that needed physiologically. Thus, nocturia (usually in the form of nocturnal polyuria) or 24-hour polyuria (in which night-time and daytime overproduction of urine are both present) can reflect systemic conditions or problems with renal tubular function.

Clinical assessment is directed at deciding firstly whether there might be an underlying medical condition of which the management needs to be optimized or which has yet to be recognized in the person affected, and secondly whether the nocturia needs treatment as a symptom in its own right. As with any other clinical presentation, clinical assessment starts with history, which usefully can be supplemented by symptom assessment questionnaires. Modern questionnaires have been validated to score symptom severity and bother for all LUTS, which makes taking the history more efficient and comprehensive. A frequency/volume chart is crucial for guiding the evaluation of underlying mechanisms. Special investigations may be needed in certain contexts.

3.2 History and examination

The presence of LUTS in the categories of storage or voiding/post-micturition needs to be ascertained. The most widely used definitions of LUTS are the standardized terms defined by ICS (Table 1.1).

Nocturia should be diagnosed if the individual has to wake at night one or more times to void [1, 2]. The term 'night-time frequency' differs from that for nocturia, as it includes voids that occur after the individual has gone to bed, but before he/she has gone to sleep, and voids which occur in the early morning which prevent the individual from getting back to sleep as he/she wishes [1]. If this definition is used, then an adapted definition of daytime frequency would need to be used with it.

The presence of a range of LUTS, in addition to nocturia, suggests lower urinary tract dysfunction may be a contributory aspect of nocturia, although additional contributory factors do still need to be considered. The presence of enuresis should be sought by questioning as to whether the patient passes urine, whilst remaining asleep, and thereby wets nightclothes and the bed. Nocturia can also be an aspect of bladder pain syndrome, so the presence of pain related to bladder filling, relieved by emptying, should be enquired after. Symptom assessment questionnaires are a time-effective means of comprehensively and systematically capturing

Table 3.1 Medications affecting urine output or sleep		
Increased urine output	**Direct lower urinary tract effects**	**Insomnia and central nervous system effects**
Diuretics	Ketamine	CNS stimulants (dexamfetamine, methylphenidate)
Calcium channel blockers	Tiaprofenic acid	Antihypertensives (alpha-blockers, beta-blockers, methyldopa)
Tetracycline	Cyclophosphamide	Respiratory (salbutamol, theophylline)
Lithium		Decongestants (phenylephrine, pseudoephedrine)
		Hormones (corticosteroids, thyroid)
		Psychotropics (MAOIs, SSRIs, atypical antidepressants)
		Dopaminergic agonists (carbidopa)
		Anti-epileptics (phenytoin)
CNS, central nervous system; MAOI, monoamine oxidase inhibitor; SSRI, selective serotonin reuptake inhibitor. (Adapted from *BJU International*, Gulur et al., Nocturia as a manifestation of systemic disease, Copyright (2011), with permission from John Wiley and Sons.)		

Initial number | ICIQ-N 01/06 | DAY MONTH YEAR

CONFIDENTIAL

Today's date

Nocturia

Many people experience urinary symptoms some of the time. We are trying to find out how many people experience urinary symptoms, and how much they bother them. We would be grateful if you could answer the following questions, thinking about how you have been, on average, over the PAST FOUR WEEKS.

1. **Please write in your date of birth:** DAY MONTH YEAR

2 **Are you** *(tick one)*: Female ☐ Male ☐

3a. How often do you pass urine during the day?

1 to 6 times ☐	0
7 to 8 times ☐	1
9 to 10 times ☐	2
11 to 12 times ☐	3
13 times or more ☐	4

3b. How much does this bother you?
Please ring a number between 0 (not at all) and 10 (a great deal)

0 1 2 3 4 5 6 7 8 9 **10**
not at all … a great deal

4a. During the night, how many times do you have to get up to urinate, on average?

none ☐	0
one ☐	1
two ☐	2
three ☐	3
four or more ☐	4

4b. How much does this bother you?
Please ring a number between 0 (not at all) and 10 (a great deal)

0 1 2 3 4 5 6 7 8 9 **10**
not at all … a great deal

Thank you very much for answering these questions.

Figure 3.1 International Consultation on Incontinence Modular Questionnaire (ICIQ) questionnaires for nocturia (ICIQ-N).

Reproduced with permission from ICIQ.net. *The Journal of Urology*, **175**(3), Abrams *et al.*, The International Consultation on Incontinence Modular Questionnaire: <http://www.iciq.net>, pp. 1063–1066, Copyright (2006).

relevant features. In the field of nocturia, there are dedicated questionnaires for nocturia severity and QoL impact. The International Consultation on Incontinence Modular Questionnaire (ICIQ) has developed specific questionnaires for nocturia (ICIQ-N) (Figure 3.1) [3] and QoL impact of nocturia (ICIQ-NQol) (Figure 3.2) [4]. These are particularly useful where nocturia is a predominant symptom.

Where other LUTS are also prominent, broader symptom assessment tools, such as the ICIQ-Male LUTS (ICIQ-MLUTS) and ICIQ-Female LUTS (ICIQ-FLUTS) tools, provide

Initial number	ICIQ-Nqol 08/04 CONFIDENTIAL	DAY MONTH YEAR Today's date

Quality of life

The following statements are about the impact of 'having to get up at night to urinate'. For each item, please **mark an (X)** in the box next to the response that best describes how you have felt. Please mark **only one box** for each statement.

1. Please write in your date of birth: DAY MONTH YEAR

2. Are you *(tick one)*: Female ☐ Male ☐

OVER THE PAST FOUR WEEKS, HAVING TO GET UP AT NIGHT TO URINATE …

3. Has made it difficult for me to concentrate the next day

every day	☐	4
most days	☐	3
some days	☐	2
rarely	☐	1
never	☐	0

4. Has made me feel generally low in energy the next day

every day	☐	4
most days	☐	3
some days	☐	2
rarely	☐	1
never	☐	0

5. Has required me to nap during the day

every day	☐	4
most days	☐	3
some days	☐	2
rarely	☐	1
never	☐	0

6. Has made me less productive the next day

every day	☐	4
most days	☐	3
some days	☐	2
rarely	☐	1
never	☐	0

Figure 3.2 International Consultation on Incontinence Modular Questionnaire (ICIQ) questionnaires for quality of life impact of nocturia (ICIQ-NQol).

(Reproduced from *Urology*, **63**(3), Abraham *et al.*, Development and validation of a quality-of-life measure for men with nocturia, pp. 481–486, Copyright (2004), with permission from Elsevier.)

an assessment of all lower urinary symptoms, rating both severity and bother. In the ICIQ-MLUTS questionnaire, the specific question related to the nocturia is 'During the night, how many times do you have to get up to urinate on average?', scored between 0 and 4. This is immediately followed by the question 'How much does this bother you?', rated from 0 to 10 ('not at all' to 'a great deal'). There is also a question 'Do you leak urine when you are asleep?', also scored from 0 to 4, and again linked to a specific bother question.

Nocturia also features in the well-known International Prostate Symptom Score (IPSS) where the relevant question is 'How many times do you typically get up at night to urinate?', scored from 0 to 5, averaged over the preceding month. For the IPSS, bother is scored globally for all LUTS, rather than for each individual LUTS. Recently, a slightly simplified questionnaire, called the 'Urgency, Weak stream, Incomplete emptying, and Nocturia' (UWIN) score, has been introduced and validated [5]. Questionnaires can also be used to assess sleep, of which the Pittsburgh Sleep Quality Index (PSQI) is a well-known example [6].

During history-taking, enquiries should be made regarding habits such as fluid intake and sleep environment. Evening intake of fluid volume, caffeinated drinks, or alcoholic beverages should be captured, and also the type and time of meals in the evening as many foods contain mainly water such as fruits, salads, and vegetables. The sleep environment should be considered, e.g. noise levels and temperature. The mental state should also be considered. Anxiety and depression can be significant contributors to difficulty sleeping. The possibility of undiagnosed underlying depression should be considered, and a simple screening measure, such as the hospital anxiety and depression scale (HADS), may be appropriate. For some patients, anxiety or depression may be precipitated by their LUTS [7]. For some patients, they may be concerned about the possibility of underlying malignancy as a cause of their LUTS. Many male patients can be concerned that prostate cancer is a factor in LUTS, and simple screening and reassurance can be a suitable measure in such cases.

The past medical history should be screened, focusing on known conditions which can be relevant in urine production. These include endocrine dysfunctions such as diabetes mellitus or diabetes insipidus. Congestive cardiac failure, renal dysfunction, pulmonary disease, and neurological disease are potentially relevant [8]. The possibility of an as yet undiagnosed medical condition should also be considered. Questions related to erectile dysfunction, shortness of breath, swelling of ankles, and nocturnal breathing interruptions may be appropriate. Additionally, a past medical history of conditions or medications affecting sleep should be considered. A list of medications which can affect urine output or sleep quality is given in Table 3.1.

Physical examination should include a general medical examination, with additional focused examination to look at the body habitus (in case of the possibility of obstructive sleep apnoea) and the abdomen to look for any abdominal or pelvic masses that are compressing the bladder or a palpable bladder or kidneys, pelvic examination, and evidence of fluid retention (dependent oedema, usually seen as swollen ankles).

Examination should also include a digital rectal examination in men and vaginal examination in women to look for prolapse, oestrogen status, anal tone and sensation, and pelvic squeeze as well as a neurological examination of the lower limbs. This may help to diagnose a neurological problem, which can be relevant in nocturia.

A cardiovascular and respiratory examination needs to be performed to rule out any congestive cardiac failure signs, especially pitting oedema of the lower limbs and any sign of wheeziness in the chest which may cause shortness of breath at night, causing the patient to rise and void.

Following this, some simple bedside tests can be performed. These include measurement of the height and weight to calculate the body mass index, and therefore help diagnose obesity which can be a factor in causing sleep apnoea. Measurement of blood pressure may help in the diagnosis of cardiac or renal problems.

3.3 Bladder diary

History alone is unreliable at cataloguing urine volumes, and a frequency/volume chart (FVC) or bladder diary measured over at least 3 days is an essential element in the assessment of nocturia [9]. The number of days that an FVC needs to be completed depends on the information required. FVCs can vary from 1-day to 14-day charts. ICS recommends that, for nocturia, an FVC has to be for 24–72 hours. However, in our opinion, 24 hours is not very informative, as nocturia may vary from day to day and depends on the individual's drinking habits, as mentioned earlier; thus, it may be worse at weekends, compared to weekdays, when some patients may drink in greater amounts, e.g. several beers on a Saturday night. Also, it may be difficult to assess other LUTS, such as daytime frequency and incontinence, with a 1-day chart.

Written instructions on an FVC are normally adequate for most patients, and intensive personal instruction is not necessary. We normally send an FVC to patients with their clinic appointment, as this saves them having to attend another clinic appointment, and they can have a diagnosis and treatment initiated sooner rather than later.

We have used a 7-day FVC until recently, as this would include weekends and weekdays, but patients sometimes had difficulty completing them, especially if they are working. We have now changed to a 3-day FVC, based on evidence that a 3-day chart gives the same information as, if not better than, a 7-day FVC. The FVC, for purposes of nocturia, should include recording the time of going to bed with the intention of sleeping and the time of rising with the intention of getting up for the day.

The FVC provides the most important objective information, as it enables the categorization of patients into those with 24-hour polyuria, nocturnal polyuria, sleep disturbance, or reduced nocturnal bladder capacity [10]. This can be differentiated easily through mathematical analysis of the chart, which can give a range of useful information (Table 3.2) [11]. The key points to note are whether there is polyuria (an overall urine output in excess of 40 mL per kg body weight per 24 hours), nocturnal polyuria (where more than a third of the 24-hour output is made during the hours of sleep), and whether there are frequent voids of small volume. The FVC can also be used to evaluate the sleep duration (Table 3.2).

Table 3.2 Parameters of nocturia derived from a frequency/volume chart (FVC)	
Parameter	Description
Actual number of nightly voids (ANV)	Night-time voids observed from the FVC
Functional bladder capacity (FBC)	Largest single recorded voided volume from the FVC (equals the maximum voided volume)
Nocturnal urine volume (NUV)	Night-time voided volumes plus first morning voided volume
Nocturia index (Ni)	NUV/FBC
Predicted number of nightly voids (PNV)	Ni − 1
Nocturnal bladder capacity index (NBCi)	ANV − PNV
Nocturnal polyuria index (NPi)	NUV/24-hour total voided volume
(Adapted from *The Journal of Urology*, **175**(3), Jeffrey Weiss, Nocturia: 'Do the Math', pp. 16–18, Copyright (2006), with permission from Elsevier.)	

NAME

DATE: ___/___/___

DAY 1

Time	Drinks		Urine output (mls)	Bladder sensation	Pads
	Amount	Type			
6am					
7am					
8am					
9am					
10am					
11am					
Midday					
1pm					
2pm					
3pm					
4pm					
5pm					
6pm					
7pm					
8pm					
9pm					
10pm					
11pm					
Midnight					
1am					
2am					
3am					
4am					
5am					

Please complete this **3 day** bladder diary. Enter the following in each column against the time. You can change the specified times if you need to. In the time column, please write **BED** when you went to bed and **WOKE** when you woke up.

Drinks Write the amount you had to drink and the type of drink.

Urine output Enter the amount of urine you passed in millilitres (mls) in the urine output column, day and night. Any measuring jug will do. If you passed urine but couldn't measure it, put a tick in this column. If you leaked urine at any time write **LEAK** here.

Bladder sensation Write a description of how your bladder felt when you went to the toilet using these codes

0 - If you had no sensation of needing to pass urine, but passed urine for "social reasons", for example, just before going out, or unsure where the next toilet is.

1 - If you had a normal desire to pass urine and no urgency.

"Urgency" is different from normal bladder feelings and is the sudden compelling desire to pass urine which is difficult to defer, or a sudden feeling that you need to pass urine and if you don't you will have an accident.

2 - If you had urgency but it had passed away before you went to the toilet.

3 - If you had urgency but managed to get to the toilet, still with urgency, but did not leak urine.

4 - If you had urgency and could not get to the toilet in time so you leaked urine.

Pads If you change a pad put a tick in the pads column.

Here is an example of how to complete the diary:

Time	Drinks		Urine output	Bladder sensation	Pads
	Amount	Type			
6am WOKE					
7am	300ml	tea	350ml	2	
8am			✓		
9am				2	
10am	cup	water	Leak	3	✓

DATE: ___/___/___

DAY 2

Time	Drinks		Urine output (mls)	Bladder sensation	Pads
	Amount	Type			
6am					
7am					
8am					
9am					
10am					
11am					
Midday					
1pm					
2pm					
3pm					
4pm					
5pm					
6pm					
7pm					
8pm					
9pm					
10pm					
11pm					
Midnight					
1am					
2am					
3am					
4am					
5am					

Bladder sensation codes

0 – No sensation of needing to pass urine, but passed urine for "social reasons"

1 – Normal desire to pass urine and no urgency

2 – Urgency but it had passed away before you went to the toilet.

3 – Urgency but managed to get to the toilet, still with urgency, but did not leak urine

4 – Urgency and could not get to the toilet in time so you leaked urine

DATE: ___/___/___

DAY 3

Time	Drinks		Urine output (mls)	Bladder sensation	Pads
	Amount	Type			
6am					
7am					
8am					
9am					
10am					
11am					
Midday					
1pm					
2pm					
3pm					
4pm					
5pm					
6pm					
7pm					
8pm					
9pm					
10pm					
11pm					
Midnight					
1am					
2am					
3am					
4am					
5am					

Figure 3.3 International Consultation on Incontinence Questionnaire Bladder Diary (ICIQ-BD).

(Adapted from *European Urology*, **66**(2), Bright *et al.*, Developing and Validating the International Consultation on Incontinence Questionnaire Bladder Diary, pp. 294–300, Copyright (2014), with permission from Elsevier.)

Table 3.3 Example of FVC analysis

Daytime(from waking up to going to bed)		Night-time(from going to bed to getting up)	
Time	Voided volume (mL)	Time	Voided volume (mL)
Time of waking up: 07.00	200	Time of going to bed: 22.05	Watching TV in bed
08.15	200	23.00	200 (Fell asleep at 23.30)
12.00	350	01.00	200
16.30	400	03.00	300
18.30	250	06.00	400
22.00	200	Woke up at 08.00 next morning and voided 200 mL	

➢ Maximum voided volume 400 mL

➢ Daytime frequency: 6 times (200, 200, 350, 400, 250, 200)

➢ Night-time frequency: 4 times (200, 200, 300, 400)

➢ Nocturia episodes: 3 times (200, 300, 400)

➢ 24-hour urine volume: 200+350+400+200+200+200+200+300+400+200=2700

➢ Nocturnal urine volume: 200+300+400+200=1100

➢ NPi: 1100/2700 = 40.7% i.e. nocturia due to nocturnal polyuria

➢ Ni: (200+300+400+200)/400 = 2.75 i.e. i.e. nocturia due to nocturnal polyuria

➢ NBCi: 3-(2.75-1) = 1.25 i.e. nocturia is probably *not* due to reduced bladder capacity

The FVC can be supplemented by additional information such as fluid intake or symptom scores [12] (Figure 3.3). It is then known as a bladder diary, according to ICS standardized terminology. Without the FVC, the diagnoses cannot be made, and therefore inappropriate treatment may be given, resulting in a waste of the patient's time and of health service resources. Thus, the FVC forms the most important and indispensable part of the evaluation of nocturia. See Table 3.3 for an example FVC analysis.

3.4 Investigations

3.4.1 Biochemical blood tests

Simple measurement of urea and electrolytes is a common assessment which can provide useful information, since chronic kidney disease can influence urine output. In modern practice, the glomerular filtration rate (GFR) is often estimated and provides a slightly more accurate assessment of renal function. If the GFR is normal, it does not exclude a renal factor in nocturia—renal tubules are the main element controlling output, and renal tubular dysfunction (e.g. nephrogenic diabetes insipidus) is not necessarily associated with abnormal urea or electrolytes (which results from glomerular dysfunction). Electrolyte levels should be reviewed. Sodium levels can be particularly relevant, since a disrupted sodium level may reflect a natriuretic component of urine output. Furthermore, treatment with desmopressin requires a normal baseline level of sodium. Abnormal protein levels or calcium levels can influence urine output. Prostate cancer has been associated with nocturia, and prostate-specific antigen (PSA) measurement after counselling may be indicated.

3.4.2 Urinalysis

This can be done using a urine 'dipstick'. If any abnormalities are found, then the urine can be sent for microscopy, culture, and sensitivity. Urinary tract infection or inflammation can contribute to increased voiding frequency, including nocturia. The presence of protein may trigger the need to assess renal function, and a spot test of protein-to-creatinine ratio can be informative for this.

3.4.3 Free flow rate and post-void residual

These assessments are conventionally undertaken in assessing LUTS. Impaired maximum flow rate points towards voiding dysfunction, and the presence of a substantial PVR is likely to increase urinary frequency, including during night time.

3.4.4 Ultrasound scan of the renal tract

An ultrasound scan to look at the renal structure and bladder emptying is not usually indicated, unless there is an abnormality on kidney function tests or urinalysis, or a significant post-void residual (PVR). Significant findings, such as renal masses, which are relevant to nocturia are unusual, but, if present, they must be identified and evaluated.

3.4.5 Urodynamic studies

These can have a role, if LUTS are clearly present in association with the patient's nocturia and conservative and medical therapy have failed in resolving the symptoms. Conventional urodynamic assessment is unable to assess specific mechanisms underlying nocturia, since the patient is not in a suitable sleeping environment when undergoing urodynamic tests. Conclusions from urodynamic studies, such as detrusor overactivity or BOO, can therefore only be regarded as indirect at best.

3.4.6 Cystoscopic examination

Cystoscopy and biopsy to look for signs of interstitial cystitis, bladder stones, or bladder cancer are not usually indicated, unless there is an abnormality on previous investigations such as blood on urinalysis.

3.5 Specialized assessment

If a specific endocrine, nephrological, neurological, or cardiovascular problem is present, specialist referral may be warranted. Sleep studies and nocturnal oximetry can be used to screen for obstructive sleep apnoea and can be useful to identify parasomnias, restless leg syndrome, and other sleep abnormalities. The presence of such abnormalities is potentially important, since they may cause the patient to wake, following which the patient may become aware of the need to pass urine. This would make the nocturia the secondary, rather than the primary, cause of sleep disturbance.

3.6 Conclusions

The clinical assessment of nocturia is focused on identifying severity and bother, and establishing various potential underlying mechanisms in order to guide treatment selection. Key information with regard to the presence of LUTS, contributory habits, and systemic medical conditions must be obtained. The use of a screening questionnaire is the most time-efficient way to obtain much of this information. Examination should be directed toward potential contributory factors. The bladder diary (FVC) is an indispensable element of the assessment. Further specific tests are guided by individual circumstances.

References

1. Abrams P, et al. (2002). The standardisation of terminology of lower urinary tract function: report from the Standardisation Sub-committee of the International Continence Society. *Neurourol Urodyn.* **21**:167–78.

2. Van Kerrebroeck P, et al. (2002). The standardization of terminology in nocturia: report from the Standardization Subcommittee of the International Continence Society. *BJU Int.* **90** Suppl 3:11–15.

3. Abrams P, Avery K, Gardener N, Donovan J (2006). The International Consultation on Incontinence Modular Questionnaire:. www.iciq.net *J Urol.* **175**(3 Pt 1):1063–6; discussion 1066.

4. Abraham L, et al. (2004). Development and validation of a quality-of-life measure for men with nocturia. *Urology.* **63**: 481–6.

5. Eid K, et al. (2014). Validation of the Urgency, Weak stream, Incomplete emptying, and Nocturia (UWIN) score compared with the American Urological Association Symptoms Score in assessing lower urinary tract symptoms in the clinical setting. *Urology.* **83**:181–5.

6. Buysse DJ, et al. (1989). The Pittsburgh Sleep Quality Index: a new instrument for psychiatric practice and research. *Psychiatry Res.* **28**:193–213.

7. Coyne KS, et al. (2009). The burden of lower urinary tract symptoms: evaluating the effect of LUTS on health-related quality of life, anxiety and depression: EpiLUTS. *BJU Int.* **103** Suppl 3:4–11.

8. Gulur DM, Mevcha AM, and Drake MJ (2011). Nocturia as a manifestation of systemic disease. *BJU Int.* **107**:702–13.

9. Bright E, Drake MJ, and Abrams P (2011). Urinary diaries: evidence for the development and validation of diary content, format, and duration. *Neurourol Urodyn.* **30**:348–52.

10. Cornu JN, et al. (2012). A contemporary assessment of nocturia: definition, epidemiology, pathophysiology, and management—a systematic review and meta-analysis. *Eur Urol.* **62**:877–90.

11. Weiss JP (2006). Nocturia: 'do the math'. *J Urol.* **175**(3 Pt 2): S16–18.

12. Bright E, et al. (2014). Developing and validating the International Consultation on Incontinence Questionnaire bladder diary. *Eur Urol.* **66**:294–300.

Chapter 4

Treatment of nocturia

Daniel P. Verges and Jeffrey P. Weiss

Key points

- Nocturia may result from several unrelated causes, and, therefore, following a detailed assessment of the patient, treatment of nocturia should be appropriate to the cause or causes.
- Initial treatment usually includes lifestyle interventions and behavioural modifications such as:
  - reducing fluid intake at least 4 hours prior to bedtime, e.g. caffeine and/or alcohol, both of which are mild diuretics
  - limiting excessive food volume intake prior to bedtime, e.g. fruits, vegetables
  - in those with dependent oedema:
    - adequate exercise
    - elevating leg in the afternoon above heart level
    - compression stockings
  - emptying bladder before going to bed.
- If conservative treatment fails to control the patient's symptoms, then medical treatment is aimed at the primary cause of the nocturia.
- Combination therapy may be required in some cases. However, high-quality clinical trials looking at these combinations are lacking.

4.1 Conservative management of nocturia

4.1.1 Lifestyle interventions and behavioural changes

It can be seen from the previous chapters that nocturia may result from several unrelated causes, and, therefore, following a detailed assessment of the patient, treatment of nocturia should be appropriate to the cause or causes. Before initiation of pharmacologic therapy for nocturia, a trial of conservative management, consisting of lifestyle modifications and behavioural changes, is warranted. These conservative measures, amongst others, include:

- voiding prior to retiring to sleep
- moderation of intake or avoidance of alcohol and caffeine (especially afternoon and evening caffeine intake)
- leg elevation above the heart level and/or use of compression stockings to mobilize fluid which has been third-spaced during wakeful activity
- fluid restriction, usually at least 4 hours preceding sleep
- practising good sleep hygiene:

- optimizing conditions for sleep via engaging in moderate exercise, paying attention to room light, noise, and temperature
- use of natural sleep aids/supplements
- use of protective undergarments/pads/diapers to decrease soiling of sleep environment in the event of nocturia causing nocturnal enuresis.

4.1.2 Evidence from studies of conservative management

Evidence supporting conservative management of nocturia includes case series, cohort studies, and a few randomized trials in men and women.

In a prospective series of 82 patients (mean age 66 ± 8.3 years, 63 men and 19 women) with polyuria (including nocturia), a 30-minute systematized behavioural modification programme was tested to assess its effect on voiding dysfunction and bother. This behavioural programme consisted of regulation of fluid intake, watching videos about normal bladder physiology and storing and emptying, and explanations with examples and counselling with a nurse practitioner. Patients could receive this training more than once if needed or indicated. The authors reported significant improvement in nocturnal voids, QoL scores, Ni, and NBCi in 78.5% of patients after the first intervention, with 13.9% of patients being dissatisfied with the results of the behavioural intervention. The authors found no additional benefit in outcomes after a second behavioural intervention [1].

In another randomized clinical trial of women with mixed urinary incontinence and nocturia ($n = 131$, age 55–93), FVC analysis was performed to compare the efficacy of pharmacotherapy with an antimuscarinic medication to behavioural modification. Behavioural modification consisted of four sessions of biofeedback/pelvic floor muscle exercises, and drug treatment consisted of oxybutynin immediate-release titrated up to a maximum of 5 mg orally three times/day. A placebo group was included, and patients were randomized between these three groups for a treatment period of 8 weeks. Upon completion of the study, behavioural therapy reduced nocturia by a median of 0.50 nocturnal voids/night, whereas pharmacotherapy reduced nocturnal voids/night by 0.30 ($p = 0.03$), and placebo reduced nocturnal voids by 0.0 episodes/night ($p < 0.001$) [2].

A randomized trial of behavioural treatment versus antimuscarinic therapy in men with BOO with persistent OAB symptoms despite alpha-blocker therapy ($n = 143$, age 42–88) also supports beginning therapy with behavioural changes. After a 4-week run-in with alpha-blocker therapy, men with persistent urinary urgency and >8 voids/day, with or without urgency incontinence, were randomized to behavioural therapy or drug therapy. Behavioural therapy consisted of pelvic floor muscle exercises, urgency, suppression and delayed voiding, and drug therapy consisted of oxybutynin extended-release titrated on an individual patient basis to between 5 and 30 mg/day. Seven-day FVCs showed that reduction of nocturia episodes was superior with behavioural therapy versus pharmacologic therapy (−0.7 versus −0.32, respectively; $p = 0.05$) [3].

A multifaceted intervention plan to reduce severity and bother of nocturia was assessed in a prospective study of 55 men (mean age 67 years) by the US Veterans Administration. FVCs and American Urological Association (AUA) symptom scores were assessed at baseline, after which patients underwent behavioural therapy and drug therapy. Study participants were given individualized behavioural intervention plans, but all study participants were asked to decrease alcohol and caffeine intake, limit evening fluids, and practise good sleep hygiene. Bladder diaries and AUA symptom index (AUA-SI; IPSS) were assessed after 4 weeks and compared to baseline values. Nocturnal voids decreased from 2.6 to 1.9 ($p < 0.001$) in 50/55 men, and the bother score was reduced from 3.1 to 1.1 ($p < 0.001$) in 53/55 men [4].

In a prospective randomized trial in women with OAB (age > 18), bladder training and drug therapy with tolterodine were compared. Bladder training consisted of pelvic floor and bladder anatomy lessons and analysis of FVCs. Patients were instructed to use timed voiding to reach an inter-void time interval of 3–4 hours and a voided volume of 300–400 mL. For 12 weeks, this training was assessed on its own and in combination with tolterodine therapy (2 mg orally twice a day). Additionally, this training was assessed compared to tolterodine alone. Post-treatment FVC analysis revealed decreased nocturia, compared to baseline, in all groups, with 56.1% decrease in the bladder training group ($p < 0.05$), 65.4% decrease in the tolterodine group ($p < 0.05$), and 66.3% decrease in the combination group ($p < 0.05$) [5]. This study provides similar evidence for tolterodine and behavioural therapy as treatments for nocturia.

Lifestyle modifications intended to decrease nocturia were assessed in a non-randomized, non-placebo-controlled evaluation in 56 patients. After assessment with FVCs, IPSS, and PSQI at baseline, the subjects restricted fluid intake, exercised daily, kept warm in bed, and avoided excessive sleep for 4 weeks, followed by repeat assessment. Average nocturnal urine volumes decreased by 155 mL (from 923 mL to 768 mL; $p = 0.0005$); nocturnal voids decreased from 3.6 to 2.7 ($p < 0.0001$), and 53.1% of subjects decreased nocturnal voids by one or more per night [6]. This study provides objective data that lifestyle modifications decrease nocturnal urine volume and nocturia, but the subjective clinical significance of this decrease may be considered questionable.

4.1.3 Summary

There is no Level 1 evidence that manipulation of fluid input helps with nocturia; however, it would be logical to assume that, if patients do not drink fluid at night before going to bed, they will fill their bladders at a slower rate, and therefore they would not have to get up to void at night, at least so often. Based on the literature (mostly consisting of Level 3 evidence), behavioural modification and changes in lifestyle can reduce both the nocturnal urine volume and the number of nocturnal voids. When used in combination with antimuscarinic therapy, in patients with overactive bladder syndrome (see Section 4.2), behavioural modification is more effective than either alone. However, it must be remembered that an objective decrease in the parameters may not necessarily translate into a clinically significant subjective improvement in patient bother scores.

Given the concern for polypharmacy in the ageing population and the increasing prevalence of nocturia as patients get older, behavioural modification should be considered first-line therapy. All patients with nocturia should reduce caffeine and alcohol intake, limit evening and night-time fluid intake, perform moderate exercise (consistent with cardiac status), and practise good sleep hygiene. Additionally, bladder training and education programmes, which may be administered by physician extenders, should also be considered, whether alone or combined with antimuscarinic medication.

After receiving advice on conservative management, patients are then advised to come back in 1–2 months for review in the outpatient clinic. They would be asked to complete a new FVC and QoL questionnaire immediately before their follow-up appointment. This allows the physician and patient to objectively and subjectively compare the pre- and post-treatment data and therefore plan further treatment, if improvement has not been adequate.

4.2 **Medical treatment of nocturia**

4.2.1 **5-alpha reductase inhibitors**

Men presenting with storage and/or emptying symptoms, such as weak urinary stream, urgency of urination, incomplete emptying, and nocturia, may be found to have prostatic enlargement and obstruction as the cause of, or a contributing factor to, this constellation of LUTS. Like alpha-blockers, 5-alpha reductase inhibitors (5-ARIs) form part of the urologist's armamentarium in the treatment of LUTS and are presumed to work by decreasing urethral resistance by reducing prostatic volume.

4.2.1.1 *Evidence for finasteride*

A systematic review of 21 945 men from 23 randomized, placebo-controlled trials was performed to assess the clinical benefits and harms of finasteride versus placebo for the treatment of LUTS due to prostatic enlargement and obstruction. The goal of the study was to assess for a meaningful change in AUA-SI/IPSS, as defined by a change greater than, or equal to, 4 points. These trials showed that there was no significant improvement in nocturia with the use of finasteride. Subgroup analysis, however, showed a significant reduction in nocturia in men aged 70 years or older ($n = 127$, -0.29 and -0.11 for drug and placebo, respectively; $p <$ 0.05). However, these small mean changes are unlikely to be clinically meaningful in most men treated by finasteride [7].

4.2.1.2 *Conclusions*

Whilst there is Level 1 evidence that 5-ARIs do not reduce nocturnal voids in men <70 years old with LUTS, finasteride does decrease the progression of benign prostatic enlargement (BPE), urinary retention, and surgical intervention for prostatic enlargement. There is some evidence that men older than 70 years of age with bothersome nocturia may benefit from 5-ARI therapy. This information is clinically useful, especially considering that the urologist of today and tomorrow will be caring for an increasingly ageing population.

4.2.2 **Selective alpha-1 adrenergic antagonists**

By decreasing bladder outlet resistance, these agents may improve emptying, and thereby reduce storage LUTS (e.g. nocturia), by increasing voided volumes. Many trials and meta-analyses have examined alpha-1 blocker therapy for the treatment of LUTS. In so doing, many have directly or indirectly evaluated the effect of alpha-1 receptor blockade on nocturia.

4.2.2.1 *Evidence for doxazosin*

In a randomized controlled trial (RCT) of men ($n = 2583$) with at least one nocturnal void at baseline being treated with doxazosin and/or finasteride, treatment was assessed via self-reported nocturia before and after intervention (at 1 and 4 years post-treatment). After 1 year, nocturia (voids/night) was reduced by 0.35 in the placebo group, 0.40 in the finasteride group ($p > 0.05$, non-significant), 0.54 in the doxazosin group ($p < 0.05$), and 0.58 ($p < 0.05$) in the combination group. At the 4-year analysis, doxazosin and combination therapy remained statistically significant, relative to placebo ($p < 0.05$). One-year follow-up secondary analysis of 495 men older than 70 years revealed that all of these drugs significantly decreased nocturnal voids (finasteride 0.29, doxazosin 0.46, and combination 0.42), compared to placebo (0.11; $p < 0.05$) [8]. Again, given significant therapeutic effect in older patients, as is the case with 5-ARIs, a one-size-fits-all approach to the treatment of nocturia is not supported by the data [8].

When three RCTs were compared in a combined cohort of 955 men with benign prostatic obstruction (BPO) treated with alpha-blocker therapy (alfuzosin, $n = 473$) versus placebo ($n = 482$), a significant net decrease of 0.3 voids per night was seen (drug minus placebo) [9].

An open-label randomized study of 189 men in China, aged between 50 and 84 years, compared nocturia treatment efficacy of doxazosin ($n = 94$) to that of tamsulosin ($n = 95$). As in many other studies, nocturia was assessed by question 7 of the IPSS and a bladder diary. Additionally, the authors assessed QoL and quality of sleep. At both 4 and 8 weeks of treatment, doxazosin significantly decreased nocturia both by IPSS question 7 analysis (for doxazosin and tamsulosin, respectively: −1.5 versus −1.1 at 4 weeks, and −2.0 versus −1.6 at 8 weeks; $p < 0.001$) and by FVC analysis (for doxazosin and tamsulosin, respectively: −1.7 versus −1.3 at 4 weeks, and −2.1 versus −1.7 at 8 weeks; $p = 0.001$). The percentages of patients reporting an improved quality of sleep (for doxazosin and tamsulosin, respectively: 43.6% versus 27.4% at 4 weeks; $p = 0.02$) and QoL (for doxazosin and tamsulosin, respectively: 2.5 versus 2.8 at 4 weeks; $p = 0.001$, and 2.1 versus 2.5 at 8 weeks; $p < 0.001$) were also improved in the doxazosin group [10]. Of note, the dose of tamsulosin used in this study, i.e. 0.2 mg, is less than the dose used in other clinical settings [10].

When secondary analysis of nocturia in 1078 male veterans with BPE, who were randomly assigned to receive terazosin, finasteride, combination, or placebo, was performed, nocturnal voids decreased from a baseline mean of 2.5 to 2.1, 1.8, 2.1, and 2.0 episodes in the placebo, terazosin, finasteride, and combination groups, respectively. Reduction of nocturia by terazosin was statistically significant, compared to combination therapy, finasteride, and placebo ($p = 0.03$, $p = 0.0001$, and $p = 0.0001$, respectively). This study shows that terazosin and combination therapy reduced the number of nocturia episodes in men with BPE. It is wise to note, however, that terazosin was only 'better' than placebo by 0.3 nocturnal voids/night. Whilst this is a statistically significant difference, it may not translate into a clinically meaningful benefit [11].

According to a post hoc data analysis in men older than 50 with symptoms of BPO, 8 mg silodosin daily was significantly more effective than either placebo or 0.4 mg tamsulosin in improving nocturia, frequency, and emptying [12].

Seven hundred and forty-four men with BPE taking naftopidil for LUTS from eight trials were studied in a systematic review to assess the effect on LUTS (including nocturia). No trial compared naftopidil (selective alpha-1-d adrenergic receptor blocker) with placebo. In 419 patients from five trials, mean improvement in IPSS of 8.4 points was seen with naftopidil versus a 8.9 point reduction in symptom score with 0.2 mg tamsulosin. Naftopidil significantly improved IPSS, with a 5.9 versus 0.4 point decrease ($p < 0.0002$) in patients on naftopidil and Eviprostat®, respectively [13]. Eviprostat® is a herbal agent which contains ethanolic extracts of umbellate wintergreen (*Chimaphila umbellata*), pasque flower (*Pulsatilla pratensis*), fresh aspen (*Populus tremula*), and horsetail (*Equisetum arvense*).

Another controlled naftopidil study randomized 59 patients with LUTS to naftopidil 50 mg ($n = 31$) or tamsulosin 0.2 mg ($n = 28$) for 6–8 weeks. The IPSS was used to rate the severity of nocturia at 2 weeks of treatment and then at the end of the study period. At 2 weeks, naftopidil, but not tamsulosin, showed significant improvement in nocturia, compared to baseline (3.5 to 2.2, $p = 0.0004$ with naftopidil versus 3.4 to 2.7, $p = 0.1$ with tamsulosin). By the end of the study period, significant improvement in nocturia was seen in both groups, with naftopidil showing a decrease in nocturia score from 3.5 to 1.6 ($p < 0.0001$) and tamsulosin yielding a 3.4 to 1.7 decrease ($p < 0.0001$) [14].

In men with LUTS previously treated with tamsulosin, naftopidil 75 mg daily significantly improved both day and night-time frequency, IPSS, and QoL index after treatment for 6 weeks. Of note, night-time frequency decreased from 3.1 (±0.6) voids per night to 1.2 (±0.8) voids per night ($p < 0.0001$) [15]. Thus, naftopidil may improve nocturia symptoms more quickly than tamsulosin.

Another alpha-1 blocker alfuzosin, given as 10 mg twice daily, was evaluated in an open-label study of 689 European men (mean age 68) over a 3-year period. At the end of the study, nocturnal voids decreased by 0.8 voids/night ($p < 0.001$) [16].

Evidence for the use of silodosin for nocturia was found in a double-blind, parallel, placebo-controlled group study of 955 patients with LUTS. Inclusion criteria were age ≥50, an IPSS ≥13, and a maximum urinary flow rate (Qmax) 4–15 mL/s. These patients were randomized to receive silodosin 8 mg ($n = 381$), tamsulosin 0.4 mg ($n = 384$), or placebo ($n = 190$)

once daily for 12 weeks. Among active treatment groups, only those in the silodosin group experienced statistically significant reduction in nocturia versus placebo ($p = 0.013$), with a change in nocturnal voids for silodosin, tamsulosin, and placebo of −0.9, −0.8, and −0.7, respectively [17].

In a prospective, non-randomized trial of 51 patients (all older than 40) with LUTS, the efficacy of tamsulosin OCAS (oral controlled absorption system—a drug formulation promoting constant drug release) was assessed over an 8-week study period. Assessment occurred at baseline and at 2, 4, and 8 weeks via the IPSS, the QoL assessment index (IPSS-QoL), and Nocturia Quality of Life (N-QoL) index. After the 8-week study period, the IPSS decreased from a baseline of 19.5 to 6.1 ($p < 0.001$), and the N-QoL improved from a baseline of 32.1 to 42.9 ($p < 0.001$) [18].

A prospective trial of 160 patients (no placebo control) with 'LUTS/BPE' and nocturia (≥2 voids/night) treated with tamsulosin for 8 weeks showed significant improvement in nocturia and in hours of undisturbed sleep. In the 97 men who showed a therapeutic response, nocturnal frequency decreased and hours of undisturbed sleep increased, as shown by FVC and IPSS analysis. The IPSS nocturia score improved from 3.1 (±1.1) before treatment to 1.8 (±0.8) after treatment ($p <0.0001$), and the FVC nocturnal voiding frequency decreased from 3.1 (±1.0) to 1.7 (±1.0) after treatment ($p < 0.0001$). Hours of undisturbed sleep improved from 2.1 (±1.0) before treatment to 3.5 (±1.5) after treatment ($p < 0.0001$). Whilst not randomized, this study provides Level 3 evidence that tamsulosin may decrease nocturnal voids and improve hours of undisturbed sleep [19].

Decreasing nocturia and increasing hours of undisturbed sleep is clinically meaningful, as reduction in nocturnal awakenings to void is associated with increasing QoL. Along these lines, in a prospective trial of 93 men with LUTS treated with 0.2 mg tamsulosin daily (mean age 70 years; non-randomized), the most significant factor in improvement of QoL was improvement of the bother score for nocturia [20].

4.2.2.2 *Conclusions*

Most of the studies that examined men with LUTS and presumed BPO utilized QoL assessments, FVCs, and symptomatic assessment via the IPSS. There is Level 1 evidence demonstrating that most selective alpha-1 adrenergic antagonists (alfuzosin, doxazosin, naftopidil, silodosin, tamsulosin, and terazosin) are more effective than placebo in decreasing nocturia in men with BPO who have nocturia.

There is Level 3 evidence that men treated with one prostate-specific agent who have failed to improve their nocturia may benefit from a trial of another agent in the same class, although it is not clear why switching to another drug in the same class should be effective, and little of the evidence comes from high-quality research. Overall, treatment effect is weak and, at best, barely exceeds a minimally identifiable threshold for patient perception of improvement.

4.2.3 **Antimuscarinic agents**

Antimuscarinic agents are used to treat overactive bladder, of which nocturia is a prominent component [21]. Through their action on muscarinic cholinergic receptors in the detrusor muscle, in the urothelium, and on bladder neurons, they decrease detrusor muscle and possible afferent neuron activity, and improve urine storage [22]. Because nocturia may be caused by diminished nocturnal functional bladder capacity, these agents have been used to treat nocturia. As with the 5-ARIs and alpha-blockers, antimuscarinics are not known to affect diurnal or nocturnal urine production; their potential therapeutic effect in patients with nocturnal polyuria is expectedly poor. Side effects of these agents are due to inhibition of cholinergic receptors and consist of dry mouth, constipation, and potential dizziness. Contraindications to their use include urinary retention, highly elevated PVR volume, and narrow-angle glaucoma. These agents should be used with caution in the frail elderly, as they may cause delirium, exacerbate dementia, or produce cognitive slowing or dysfunction.

4.2.3.1 *Evidence for tolterodine*

A double-blind, placebo-controlled trial ($n = 745$) evaluated 4 mg tolterodine extended release (tolterodine-ER) given at bedtime (<4 hours before retiring) versus placebo for the treatment of nocturia in men over a study period of 12 weeks. Mean age was 64 years old; 374 men were randomized to placebo, and 371 were randomized to tolterodine-ER. Data were collected in the form of FVC and urinary urgency rating for each void. The urgency scale was ranked on a scale of 1 to 5: 1 = no urgency, 2 = mild urgency, 3 = moderate urgency, 4 = severe urgency, 5 = urgency incontinence. OAB was defined as an urgency scale score of 3–5, and severe OAB was defined as a score of 4–5. Post hoc analysis, after the 12-week study period, showed a statistically significant improvement in mean night-time urgency score for the tolterodine-ER group (−0.17), compared to the placebo group (−0.03; $p < 0.01$). Daytime and 24-hour urgency was also significantly decreased. With regard to nocturnal frequency, patients with severe OAB had a significant reduction, relative to placebo (−77% for tolterodine-ER and −50% for placebo; $p < 0.01$) [23].

Another RCT allocated 850 patients, all of whom had over 8 micturitions/24 hours and nocturia (mean nocturnal voids = 2.5) ± urgency incontinence, to 4 mg tolterodine-ER or placebo within 4 hours of retiring to sleep. Over the 12-week study period, tolterodine-ER significantly reduced OAB-related nocturnal micturitions versus placebo. However, it did not significantly reduce the total number of nocturnal voids and did not affect nocturnal micturitions not due to OAB (e.g. those due to nocturnal polyuria) [24].

4.2.3.2 *Evidence for fesoterodine*

Another antimuscarinic medication fesoterodine was seen to be useful in reducing nocturnal voids, in addition to reducing other OAB symptoms, in an open-label study of 516 adults with OAB. OAB in this study was defined as greater than, or equal to, eight voids and three urgency episodes per day. Over a 12-week period, patients were treated with 4 mg fesoterodine/day. Fifty per cent of subjects had an increase in dosage by week 4 of the study period. In this study group, with treatment, nocturnal voids decreased from an average of 2.6 voids/night to 1.8 voids/night, but again there was no placebo comparator [25].

Other Level 1 evidence, however, does not suggest a significant fesoterodine-induced reduction in nocturnal voids. A multicentre, double-blind, and placebo- and active-controlled trial of 1135 patients with OAB symptoms randomized subjects to placebo, fesoterodine 4 mg daily, fesoterodine 8 mg daily, or tolterodine-ER 4 mg daily for 12 weeks. The percentage change in nocturnal voids for placebo alone was −26.8%, and there was no significant decrease in nocturnal voids in any of the therapeutic arms, relative to placebo: fesoterodine 4 mg (−28.6%; $p = 0.982$), fesoterodine 8 mg (−23.1%; $p = 0.896$), and tolterodine-ER 4 mg (−25%; $p = 0.815$) [26]. Further negative studies with regard to the efficacy of fesoterodine for nocturia are listed in the References section [27–29].

4.2.3.3 *Evidence for solifenacin*

A pooled analysis of four RCTs, in which patients were randomized to solifenacin 5 mg, solifenacin 10 mg, or placebo, assessed the reduction in nocturnal voids using solifenacin. Of the 3032 subjects in the combined study population, 83.5% of subjects ($n = 2534$) reported nocturia. Voiding diary analysis revealed nocturnal polyuria in 62% of the study population with nocturia. In the proportion of patients without nocturnal polyuria, there was a −0.18 nocturnal void reduction versus placebo, but, in those with nocturnal polyuria, there was no significant reduction in nocturia episodes. Further analysis of the data suggests that a high performance of placebo in reducing nocturnal voids may have caused the failure to achieve statistically significant decreased nocturia in the nocturnal polyuria group [30].

4.2.3.4 *Evidence for trospium chloride*

In a multicentre, double-blind RCT of 658 patients with average baseline nocturnal voids of twice/night, randomized to placebo versus trospium chloride 20 mg twice daily, there was a significant decrease in nocturnal voids with the use of anticholinergic medication over the 12-week study period. The change in mean nocturnal voids was −0.57 for trospium versus −0.29 for placebo [31].

In another trospium study, 523 patients were randomized to receive trospium 20 mg orally twice daily versus placebo in a parallel, double-blind RCT over 12 weeks. Voiding diaries showed that those subjects randomized to the active therapy group had decreased total daily voids, decreased urgency and incontinence, and increased voided volumes. At 12 weeks, there was noted to be a decrease in nocturia episodes of −0.47 for trospium versus −0.29 for placebo ($p < 0.05$) [32].

Trospium extended release (trospium-ER) also showed significant reduction in nocturia episodes versus placebo, with a mean nocturia episode reduction of −0.8 versus −0.6 ($p = 0.006$) [33]. The clinical significance of this benefit would appear to be marginal.

4.2.3.5 *Conclusions*

Nocturia is associated with OAB and may be the most bothersome facet of this symptom complex. There is Level 1 evidence that antimuscarinic agents can reduce nocturnal micturitions, compared to placebo. Whilst this is true, these agents seem to perform less well in mitigating non-OAB-associated nocturnal voids. With this in mind, men with nocturia and moderate to severe OAB symptoms may be offered antimuscarinic therapy after a full discussion of associated risks, benefits, and alternatives. The overall benefit of this class of medications in treating nocturia appears to be slight.

4.2.4 **Combination therapy**

For some patients, the decrease in LUTS provided by one agent may not be clinically significant, and the addition of another agent may be required. Whilst many patients suffering from nocturia are older individuals on a number of medications for chronic illnesses, combination therapy may be the key to symptom amelioration. Concern for potential polypharmacy notwithstanding, the following combinations may be considered:

- antimuscarinic medication plus alpha-1 adrenergic blockade
- 5-ARI and alpha-1 adrenergic antagonist (in selective alpha-1 adrenergic antagonists)
- alpha-1 adrenergic antagonist and phosphodiesterase-5 inhibitor (PDE5i).

4.2.4.1 *Antimuscarinic medication combined with alpha-1 adrenergic antagonist*

Level 1 evidence for this combination can be found in a 12-week placebo-controlled, double-blind RCT ($n = 879$) which compared 4 mg tolterodine-ER ($n = 217$), 0.4 mg tamsulosin ($n = 215$), and the combination of tolterodine-ER plus tamsulosin ($n = 225$) to placebo ($n = 222$). Statistically significant reduction of nocturnal voids was seen in the combination therapy group versus placebo (−0.59 versus −0.39, respectively; $p = 0.02$) [34].

A smaller RCT of 69 patients with LUTS treated over 6 weeks with either 2 mg terazosin daily ($n = 36$) or 2 mg terazosin daily plus 2 mg tolterodine twice daily ($n = 33$) also showed benefit with a combined therapeutic approach. As in many other LUTS studies, the IPSS (especially the storage symptom score) was used to compare groups. In the terazosin only group, pretreatment IPSS was 18.5 (±3.2), and post-treatment IPSS was 17.3 (±4.1) ($p = 0.033$).

In the combination group, pretreatment IPSS was 19.0 (±3.0), and post-treatment IPSS was 14.0 (±4.2) ($p < 0.001$). Thus, in this small RCT, combination therapy resulted in a lower post-treatment IPSS, and subjectively patients complained of less urgency, frequency, and nocturia after terazosin plus tolterodine versus tolterodine alone [35].

4.2.4.2 *5-alpha reductase inhibitor plus selective alpha-1 adrenergic antagonist*

The Medical Therapy of Prostate Symptoms Trial (MTOPS) assessed men with BPE and LUTS by randomizing them to placebo versus doxazosin, finasteride, or a combination of finasteride and doxazosin. In this study, 2583 men completed over 12 months of follow-up and were evaluated via self-reported symptoms of nocturia. Similar to other nocturia studies, placebo treatment decreased the mean number of nocturia episodes (by 0.35 in the current study). Doxazosin alone decreased nocturnal voids by 0.54 ($p <0.05$) and finasteride by 0.40 ($p > 0.05$) after 1 year of treatment. Combination therapy with the two active agents reduced nocturia by 0.58 ($p < 0.05$) over the same time period. Thus, both doxazosin and combination therapy showed significantly greater improvement in nocturia, compared to placebo alone [8].

4.2.4.3 *Alpha-1 adrenergic antagonist and phosphodiesterase-5 inhibitor*

In addition to their beneficial effects with regard to erectile function, PDE5is may also decrease LUTS in men with BPO. A study analysing the effect of alfuzosin, sildenafil, or a combination of these agents in men showed a decrease in LUTS in all treatment groups. Only combination therapy and alfuzosin groups showed statistically significant improvement in nocturia, urinary frequency, PVR, and maximum urinary flow. From baseline nocturia frequency, as assessed per voiding diary analysis, sildenafil decreased nocturia by 19.2% ($p = 0.40$), alfuzosin by −37.9% ($p = 0.01$), and combination therapy by −41.9% ($p = 0.003$) [36].

4.2.4.4 *Conclusions*

Level 1 evidence exists for the combination of alpha-1 adrenergic antagonists and 5-ARIs for the treatment of LUTS, including nocturia. Combination therapy may be more effective than either drug used in isolation. Similarly, RCT data support the use of antimuscarinic medication in combination with an alpha-1 adrenergic blocker, as it significantly reduces the number of nocturnal micturitions, when compared to placebo. Level 3 evidence suggests that alpha-blockers may be more effective at improving nocturia when given with a PDE5i.

Thus, men with LUTS and suspected BPO may be offered treatment with alpha-1 adrenergic antagonists combined with 5-ARIs, antimuscarinic drugs (in men with nocturia associated with other OAB symptoms), and PDE5is (in men with concomitant erectile dysfunction).

4.2.5 **Antidiuretic pharmacotherapy**

Whilst nocturia may be related to excessive fluid intake and/or OAB, excessive nocturnal urine production may play a greater role. This condition nocturnal polyuria exists when a patient excretes >33% of his or her 24-hour urine output during sleeping hours (in non-elderly patients, the proportional cut-off value for nocturnal urine production/24-hour volume decreases with age) [37]. In fact, nocturnal polyuria is seen in 72–85% of women and in 79–90% of men screened for inclusion in nocturia trials [38, 39]. Hence, control of nocturnal urine production becomes a rational therapeutic target in this group of patients [40].

Nocturnal polyuria is thought to be due, in part, to increased secretion of atrial natriuretic peptide, decreased secretion of antidiuretic hormone, or a combination of these two processes [40]. These hormones have become targets in the therapy of nocturia. Desmopressin, a synthetic analogue of AVP, retains its antidiuretic properties but does not act as a vasopressor. Whilst not approved in the United States by the Food and Drug Administration (FDA) or in the United Kingdom, desmopressin is approved for treatment of nocturia in adults in approximately 100 countries worldwide.

Desmopressin is also indicated for the treatment of central diabetes insipidus and paediatric nocturnal enuresis. Formulations of desmopressin include:

• desmopressin tablet 0.1 mg orally in the evening (may be titrated up to 0.4 mg orally for desired effect)

• desmopressin lyophilisate (MELT) 60 micrograms sublingual in the evening (may be titrated up to 240 micrograms orally for desired effect); 25–100 micrograms of MELT preparation recently approved in Canada for nocturia.

The most serious potential complication of desmopressin administration is hyponatraemia, which may be managed by close monitoring of serum sodium levels, particularly in the most susceptible patients (women, elderly, patients with low-normal serum sodium at baseline, and those with impaired renal function) [39].

4.2.5.1 *Evidence for desmopressin*

Desmopressin has been shown to provide successful treatment of nocturnal polyuria and nocturia related to underlying disease syndromes such as multiple sclerosis and Parkinson's disease. Desmopressin has been shown to increase the duration of the first sleep period before awakening to void, to decrease the frequency of nocturnal voids, and to decrease nocturnal urine production in a meta-analysis and systematic review of eight RCTs with $n = 619$ [41].

A 3-month, double-blind, placebo-controlled RCT of 261 women, aged 19–87, compared low-dose desmopressin (25 micrograms orally disintegrating tablet) to placebo for the treatment of nocturia. Mean decrease in nocturnal voids was -0.22 voids ($p = 0.028$), and the odds ratio (OR) of achieving a 33%, or greater, decrease in nocturia was 1.85 ($p = 0.006$).

Both placebo and active drug therapy groups were monitored for adverse effects, and serum sodium levels were monitored during the study period. In this trial, desmopressin was well tolerated, and serum sodium levels remained >125 mmol/L throughout the study. In this study, desmopressin increased the duration of the first sleep period by an average of 49 min, compared to placebo ($p = 0.003$). Desmopressin also significantly increased the OR of achieving a 33%, or greater, decrease in nocturia (OR 1.85, $p = 0.006$) [39].

In an RCT of men with nocturia, desmopressin orally disintegrating tablets at 50 and 75 micrograms were compared to placebo for the treatment of nocturia. Success was again defined as a 33%, or greater, decrease in nocturia. Serum sodium levels were monitored, and the groups were monitored for adverse effects. Upon final analysis, in 385 men (aged 20–87) randomized to placebo or active therapy, desmopressin increased the OR of achieving a >33% decrease in nocturia by OR 1.98 ($p = 0.0009$) and OR 2.04 ($p = 0.0004$) for desmopressin 50 micrograms and 75 micrograms, respectively. Desmopressin also significantly decreased the number of nocturnal voids, compared to placebo, by -0.37 ($p < 0.0001$) and -0.41 ($p = 0.0003$) for 50 and 75 micrograms, respectively. Desmopressin was well tolerated, with only two subjects (both older than 70) on the 50 microgram, and nine subjects on the 75 microgram, desmopressin dose having a serum sodium <130 mmol/L [38].

In the NOCTUPUS desmopressin tablet trials, 1003 patients (519 men and 484 women) were enrolled to study the safety and efficacy of desmopressin for the treatment of nocturia. Efficacy was assessed with the use of FVCs, and 157 subjects were eliminated due to non-compliance with FVC completion. Of the remaining 846 patients, after 3 weeks of therapy, 33% of men and 46% of women had a significant reduction in nocturnal voids versus placebo (significant decrease being defined as >50% reduction in nocturnal voids). In an extension study from the original NOCTUPUS trials, 67% of men and women had >50% reduction in nocturnal voids, compared to placebo [40].

Escalating doses of 10, 25, 50, or 100 micrograms of sublingual desmopressin versus placebo were studied in a 1-month-long, double-blind RCT of 757 men and women with nocturia. There were significant reductions in mean nocturnal voids for the 50 and 100 microgram doses of desmopressin, compared with placebo (-0.32, $p = 0.02$; and -0.57, $p < 0.0001$, respectively). Clinically significant hyponatraemia, defined as serum sodium <125 mmol/L, occurred in seven subjects (four women, three men) aged >65. Thus, desmopressin is largely well tolerated, but elderly and female patients appear to be more susceptible than younger patients and men to hyponatraemia [42].

4.2.5.2 *Conclusions*

The International Consultation on Incontinence have given desmopressin a Level 1 evidence and Grade A recommendation in the treatment of nocturia and nocturnal polyuria in adults <65 years old, and a Grade B recommendation in those over 65, mainly due to the increased risk of hyponatraemia. Clinically significant hyponatraemia (serum sodium <125 mmol/L) is rare but is commoner in the elderly (>65) and in women. Serial sodium testing is paramount to prevent the development of serious hyponatraemia in patients treated with desmopressin.

In patients with excessive nocturnal urine production, desmopressin may decrease both nocturnal urine production and frequency of nocturnal voids. Desmopressin is essentially safe to use in patients under 65 years old and is the treatment of choice in those with nocturnal polyuria and normal total urine production. In patients older than 65 years, it is important to ensure that the baseline urine output is <30 mL/kg/day and that baseline serum sodium levels are >135 mmol/L before administering desmopressin. Desmopressin has been licensed in several countries around the world for the treatment of nocturia. However, it is not licensed for use in patients over 65 years old but, if clinically indicated, should be used with caution under close medical supervision. Serum sodium levels need to be checked before starting treatment, and at 3 and 7 days after starting treatment or changing the dose, to help detect hyponatraemia and prevent water intoxication. We suggest serum sodium levels are also checked at 3 weeks, 3 months, 6 months, 1 year, and then yearly thereafter after being on a stable dose of desmopressin.

4.2.6 **Diuretic pharmacotherapy**

Timed diuretic pharmacotherapy may be used strategically to diurese patients prior to sleeping hours to decrease nocturia. If patients with nocturia are taking diuretics for other medical conditions, such as hypertension or congestive heart failure, then the time that these agents are ingested can be modified or optimized to decrease nocturia, e.g. administering these agents in the afternoon, as opposed to in the morning or before bedtime.

4.2.6.1 *Evidence*

The evidence-based literature supporting diuretic therapy for nocturia is sparse and consists mostly of small series and trials. In a double-blind, randomized cross-over study, late afternoon bumetanide was compared with placebo for the treatment of nocturia. Twenty-eight patients (13 females, 15 males) with at least two nocturnal voids were randomized to receive 1 mg bumetanide (a loop diuretic) or placebo over a 2-week treatment period. Bumetanide did not decrease nocturia in the ten men with a history of BOO due to BPE. In the remaining 18 patients, weekly nocturnal voids decreased by 4, relative to placebo, representing a 28% reduction in nocturia [43].

Another double-blind trial of 49 men aged >50 years with nocturnal polyuria randomized groups to receive 40 mg furosemide (a loop diuretic) or placebo 6 hours prior to sleep. Forty-three men completed the study. There was a significant reduction in nocturnal voided volume of −18% in men treated with furosemide versus −0% in men on placebo ($p < 0.001$). Additionally, the reduction in nocturia episodes was statistically significant with a decrease of 0.5 voids on average versus no decrease with placebo ($p = 0.014$). This study provides rather weak evidence that men with nocturnal polyuria may benefit from diuretic therapy 6 hours prior to sleep [44].

4.2.6.2 *Conclusions*

Loop diuretics may be useful in decreasing nocturnal voided volumes and nocturia episodes. Bumetanide may not be beneficial in men with BPO. Patients already taking diuretics for concomitant health problems may be counselled to take their diuretic medications 6 hours prior to retiring to sleep. Patients must be counselled regarding the off-label use of diuretics for nocturia.

4.2.7 **Combination of diuretic and antidiuretic**

The general advice for patients taking desmopressin is to reduce fluid input 1 hour before taking the medication to reduce the risk of hyponatraemia. Therefore, it would seem logical that patients should be given a diuretic 6 hours before going to sleep to help remove any excess fluid in the body and reduce the risk of hyponatraemia, and then have an antidiuretic at bedtime to help reduce urine production overnight.

This has been only studied in one 3-week double-blind RCT of furosemide and desmopressin versus placebo. Patients aged over 60 had at least two voids per night. There was a significant reduction in the mean number of nocturnal voids (43% versus 9%, 3.5 versus 2.0; $p < 0.01$) and nocturnal urine volume (37% versus 5%, 919.6 mL versus 584.2 mL; $p < 0.01$), with an increase in the mean duration of hours of undisturbed sleep (52% versus 19%, 133.6 min versus 203.2 min; $p < 0.01$).

4.2.8 **Botulinum toxin**

Onabotulinum toxin A is approved for refractory OAB, and there is some thinking that, in those patients with nocturia, due to failure to store urine, cystoscopic treatment with onabotulinum toxin A may alleviate nocturia. Strong evidence for the use of botulinum toxin for nocturia is limited, and most studies consist of small trials and case series which are not placebo-controlled.

In a case series of nine patients (mean age 55.8 years, mean duration of symptoms 5.5 years) with OAB and chief components of bother due to daytime frequency and nocturia, 11 cystoscopic onabotulinum toxin A injections were performed. Treatment effect was assessed with FVCs. Daytime frequency decreased by 50.8%, and nocturia decreased by 64.2%. Voided volumes also increased after treatment [45].

Onabotulinum toxin A efficacy was also assessed in a case series of ten men with 'LUTS suggestive of BPE' who had failed 6 months of medical therapy. The subjects received varying doses of onabotulinum toxin A, and LUTS were assessed before and after intervention. The mean number of nocturia events in this series decreased from 4.1 ± 0.87 pre-injection to 2.4 ± 0.84 post-injection ($p < 0.001$) [46].

4.2.8.1 *Conclusions*

Based on its mechanism of action, onabotulinum toxin A is not expected to decrease nocturia in patients with nocturnal polyuria. There is Level 3 evidence that onabotulinum toxin A can significantly reduce nocturnal micturitions in patients who have failed oral medical therapy.

The therapeutic effect of onabotulinum toxin A is transient, and injections must be repeated every 3 months. Patients must be willing to perform self-catheterization, if necessary, as urinary retention is a possible side effect of this therapy.

4.2.9 Non-steroidal anti-inflammatory agents

Anecdotally, patients may remark that their LUTS (including nocturia) are improved after taking a non-steroidal anti-inflammatory drug (NSAID) for a minor ache or pain. In fact, some patients regularly self-medicate with these agents prior to bed to decrease nocturia. These agents decrease pain through their inhibition of prostaglandin synthesis. Theoretically, by inhibiting pain signals, these agents may improve storage symptoms and decrease LUTS. Furthermore, NSAIDs may also decrease total and nocturnal urine production via decreasing the GFR, as prostaglandins normally act to dilate the afferent arteriole of the glomerulus to increase the GFR. Finally, NSAIDs may inhibit prostaglandin E2-related inhibition of antidiuretic hormone action and function as an antidiuretic [47]. Loxoprofen sodium, an NSAID, was studied over 12 months for the treatment of nocturia, as part of a multidrug regimen. Two treatment groups were assessed. Group I was treated with an alpha-blocker, a 5-ARI, and 60 mg loxoprofen before sleep. Group II received an alpha-blocker and a 5-ARI before sleep. Subjects in each group were evaluated at 3, 6, and 12 months. At the 3-month analysis, nocturia had decreased in groups I and II, but the decrease was more significant in group I (NSAID therapy) (change in nocturnal voids of -1.5 ± 0.9 and -1.1 ± 0.9 for groups I and II, respectively; $p = 0.034$). At 6 and 12 months, there was no significant difference between the groups, i.e. the apparent benefit of NSAID therapy disappeared. Based on these findings, NSAIDs may be used for limited periods to treat or augment treatment for nocturia, but they should not be used for longer than 3 months, owing to the potential for significant adverse side effects [48].

Another NSAID celecoxib was assessed for the treatment of nocturia in a double-blind, placebo-controlled RCT in men with LUTS/nocturia and BPE ($n = 80$). Men were randomized to receive 100 mg celecoxib versus placebo at 9 p.m. for 1 month. In the active drug therapy group, NSAID treatment decreased nocturnal voids from 5.17 ± 2.1 voids/night to 2.5 ± 1.9 voids/night ($p < 0.0001$). IPSS ($\pm$ standard deviation, SD) also decreased from 18.2 ± 3.4 to 15.5 ± 4.2 ($p < 0.0001$) after treatment with celecoxib. The control group did not enjoy significant decreases in nocturnal voiding frequency or IPSS values; nocturnal voids changed from 5.30 ± 2.4 before placebo administration to 5.12 ± 1.9 after placebo ($p > 0.05$), and IPSS ($\pm$ SD) changed from 18.4 ± 3.1 to 18 ± 3.9 after placebo ($p > 0.05$). Treatment effect was statistically significantly different between the randomized groups ($p < 0.0001$) [49].

4.2.9.1 Conclusions

Loxoprofen sodium may reduce nocturia for up to 3 months, but the treatment effect disappears, relative to placebo, over time, and long-term use places patients at risk of adverse events. Celecoxib appears to reduce nocturia in men with BPE. Due to the paucity of evidence and the potential for severe adverse effects with NSAID therapy, these agents cannot be recommended as first-line therapy. Patients already taking these agents for nocturia should be counselled on the existing evidence and regarding the potential for haematologic effects, gastrointestinal side effects, and increased risk of adverse cardiovascular events.

4.2.10 Oestrogens

Local vaginal oestrogens in post-menopausal women have been used in uncontrolled trials, with some benefit after 6 months' therapy.

4.3 **Surgical interventions for nocturia**

Resection of obstructing adenomatous prostatic tissue (BPO) to reduce BOO remains the gold standard for severe, bothersome LUTS. Since nocturia is often one of the most bothersome LUTS, it is reasonable to inquire as to the efficacy of surgical intervention for nocturia. A myriad of surgical options for LUTS exists on a spectrum of invasiveness and efficacy and includes simple open prostatectomy, transurethral resection of the prostate (TURP), transurethral needle ablation (TUNA), high-intensity focused ultrasound (HIFU), visual laser ablation of the prostate (VLAP), transurethral electrosurgical vaporization of the prostate (TUVP), transurethral microwave therapy (TUMT), and transurethral incision of the prostate (TUIP).

These procedural interventions have been studied to relieve BPO and LUTS, but few studies have specifically examined the role of surgery in alleviating nocturia. Some authors argue that, in performing surgery to reduce BOO, not only are LUTS improved, but PVR volume is also decreased, which may increase the time to the first nocturnal void and therefore decrease nocturia [50].

A cohort of 1258 men with LUTS was treated with watchful waiting, alpha-blocker therapy, TURP, and TUMT, and improvement in nocturia, as related to health-related QoL, was studied over a follow-up period of 6–12 months. Retrospective analysis of men in each treatment group yielded a reduction in nocturnal voids of 7%, 17%, 32%, and 75% for watchful waiting, alpha-blocker therapy, TUMT, and TURP, respectively [51].

Various surgical treatments for BPO (TUNA, HIFU, VLAP, and TUVP) were assessed in a prospective, non-randomized trial of 95 men for 6 weeks. For VLAP, there was no significant improvement in nocturia, with baseline average nocturnal voids of 4.2/night and 3.6/night after treatment. The remaining treatments did significantly improve nocturia, with a change in nocturia episodes of 3.8 to 1.2 for TURP, 2.5 to 1.3 for HIFU, 2.6 to 1.2 for TUNA, and 3.8 to 1.3 for TUVP [52].

Another study of 66 men with LUTS due to BPO (mean age of 68.9 years) randomized men to 0.4 mg tamsulosin orally once a day or TURP for alleviation of nocturia [53]. Follow-up data were assessed via IPSS, ICIQ-N (International Consultation on Incontinence Questionnaire Nocturia), and ICIQ-NQoL prior to treatment and at 3 months and 1 year post-intervention. Nocturnal awakenings were significantly decreased in the TURP group, relative to the drug therapy group. Both treatments increased hours of uninterrupted sleep (HUS), but there was no significant difference in this increase between groups.

4.3.1 **Conclusions**

Surgical therapies to reduce BOO may reduce nocturnal voids. Tamsulosin is not as effective as TURP for the treatment of BPO-related nocturia. It is important to remember that these studies were conducted in good surgical candidates who had failed medical therapy. Surgical treatments for nocturia should not be performed in the absence of prior extensive evaluation for the cause of the patient's nocturia. The studies explained should not be generalized to patients with a sole complaint of nocturia without other symptoms suggestive of BPO. Finally, patients should be advised that these procedures do not guarantee success and that nocturia may persist after surgery.

4.4 **Phytotherapy**

The supplement business is a multibillion-dollar-per-year industry which is almost entirely unregulated by the FDA. Many patients utilize a myriad of substances, whether natural or synthetic, to self-medicate an actual or perceived disease or in an attempt to optimize an already good state of health.

In fact, whilst herbal supplement manufacturers claim that their products are not intended to diagnose, treat, or cure disease, many herbal supplements are marketed for prostate health and for treating BPO. Clinicians may come across the following substances in their interactions with patients (note this is not an exhaustive or all-inclusive list):

- *Serenoa repens*, Sabal serrulata: commonly known as American dwarf palm/saw palmetto berry
- *Pygeum africanum*: the African plum tree
- *Hypoxis rooperi*: also known as South African star grass
- *Urtica dioica*: the stinging nettle
- *Secale cereale*: commonly known as rye grass/rye pollen
- *Cucurbita pepo*: pumpkin seed.

One of the most popular agents for 'prostate health' is saw palmetto [54]. This agent is widely used, despite a lack of evidence for its efficacy.

In a Cochrane systematic review of 17 RCTs (n = 2008), saw palmetto use for LUTS due to 'benign prostatic hyperplasia (BPH)/BPE' as monotherapy was evaluated. A meta-analysis showed that saw palmetto was no better than placebo in reducing LUTS, based on AUA-SI/IPSS (weighted mean difference (WMD) of −0.16 points, 95% confidence interval (CI) of −1.45 to 1.14) and Qmax (WMD 0.40 mL/s, 95% CI −0.30 to 1.09). Specifically, saw palmetto did not improve nocturia, compared to placebo (p = 0.19). This relationship held true even at double and triple the normal dose of this supplement [55].

Another systematic review of 30 RCTs comprising 5222 men analysed the effect of saw palmetto on all LUTS, including nocturia. Saw palmetto was well tolerated, but there was no significant difference in nocturia in those patients on this agent versus placebo (WMD −0.31 nightly voids; p > 0.05). When compared to finasteride, there was no advantage to saw palmetto ingestion with regard to nocturia (mean difference −0.05; p > 0.05). The same was true when compared to tamsulosin (percentage improvement of risk ratio = 0.91; p > 0.05) [54].

A double-blind, multicentre RCT of 369 men (aged 45 and greater, with Qmax >4 mL/s and AUA-SI between 8 and 24) assessed saw palmetto extract versus placebo for the treatment of LUTS (including nocturia). Even with a dose escalation at 6 and 12 months of follow-up, no treatment difference in nocturia was seen between saw palmetto and placebo [56].

Evidence for the benefit of use of the African plum tree for LUTS and nocturia is similarly lacklustre. A systematic review of 18 RCTs consisting of 1562 men being treated with *Pygeum africanum* for LUTS/nocturia versus placebo showed no statistically significant treatment difference between active supplement therapy and placebo. However, men taking *Pygeum africanum* did report a non-significant 19% reduction in nocturia (WMD −0.9 nocturnal voids; p > 0.05) [55].

Rye grass/rye pollen (*Secale cereale*) may be formulated into the herbal supplement Cernilton®. In a systematic review of the efficacy of Cernilton® on LUTS in men with 'BPE', Cernilton® was more effective in reducing nocturia than both placebo and another prostatic supplement Paraprost (L-glutamic acid–L-alanine–glycine). In this review, the weighted risk ratio for reduction in nocturia was 2.05 (95% CI 1.41 to 3.00), i.e. those taking Cernilton® were twice as likely as those taking placebo to reduce nocturnal voids. When compared to Paraprost for decreasing nocturia episodes per evening, the WMD was −0.40 voids/night (95% CI −0.73 to −0.07 voids/night). Whilst a systematic review tends to represent high-level evidence, the studies included in this analysis have been criticized for the short duration of follow-up, low numbers, differing formulations of supplements, and lack of comparison to the active control group [57]. This fact must be considered before suggesting *Secale cereale* to all patients with nocturia.

4.4.1 **Conclusions**

It is important to realize that many patients do not consider neutraceuticals to be medications. As such, physicians should specifically inquire as to the use of herbal supplement or vitamin use during the history and physical examination. Level 1 evidence suggests that saw palmetto does not represent an effective therapy for nocturia, when compared to placebo and active drug therapy. Non-significant reductions in nocturia have been shown for *Pygeum africanum* in some studies. Cernilton® may be offered or discussed with patients being treated for nocturia, given the available evidence.

4.5 **Soporific agents**

When addressing nocturia, the astute clinician attempts to verify whether it is the need to void that awakens the patient or whether the primary issue is poor sleep quality resulting in a nocturnal convenience void. When the clinician suspects the latter, he or she may consider pharmacologic agents to promote sleep, in addition to implementing good sleep hygiene measures.

In an RCT, oxazepam, a benzodiazepine, was shown to decrease nocturia severity by 63%, but there was no change in the nocturnal urine volume [58]. Thus, these agents are not expected to treat the underlying pathology in patients with nocturnal polyuria (a significant proportion of patients). Sedative agents may be useful in that they improve the return to sleep after each nocturnal void, rather than decreasing the nocturnal void frequency [59]. Of course, these agents may disturb the normal sleep architecture and may be associated with tachyphylaxis, dependence, and morning drowsiness and confusion. As such, patients should be counselled as to the risks and benefits of sedative use, and these agents should not be used with abandon.

Melatonin is a naturally occurring endocrine hormone produced by the pineal gland which is involved in the regulation of the circadian rhythm. This agent is available commercially and is used as a supplement to improve sleep quality and duration. Melatonin has a lower risk of adverse side effects, when compared to benzodiazepine medications. When given at bedtime to men with nocturia and BPE, nocturnal voids decreased by one void per night, but in a non-significant fashion, compared to placebo [60]. When compared to the hypnotic agent rilmazafone in elderly patients with nocturia, melatonin and rilmazafone decreased the number of nocturnal voids [61].

4.5.1 **Conclusions**

Whilst soporific agents may not directly address the pathophysiology of nocturia, whether due to BPO, OAB, or nocturnal polyuria, they may be used to promote quick return to sleep after a nocturnal void. Hypnotic agents are potentially habit-forming and may cause morning drowsiness or confusion. Melatonin may decrease the number of nocturnal voids, with a lower risk of adverse effects when compared to hypnotic medications.

4.6 **The future of treatment of nocturia**

At the end of the day, nocturia remains a poorly understood malady. The body of the nocturia literature is largely composed of low- to intermediate-quality evidence, and further well-designed, well-executed RCTs are necessary to verify or disprove the reported treatment effects of behavioural, medical, and surgical therapies for nocturia. Whilst

Table 4.1 Causes of, and treatment for, nocturia	
Cause of nocturia	Treatment
Overactive bladder syndrome	Antimuscarinics; onabotulinum toxin type A sacral nerve stimulation
Benign prostatic obstruction	Alpha-blockers; 5-alpha reductase inhibitors; endoscopic prostate surgery
Nocturnal polyuria	Desmopressin; furosemide
Global polyuria	Refer to medical specialist
Sleep disturbances	Refer to sleep specialist

some of the results shown in the studies are statistically significant, their clinical significance in terms of absolute reduction in nocturnal voids and, more importantly, reduction of bother and improvement in QoL may be less impressive. Combination treatment with the medications discussed may be required to treat nocturia of multiple aetiology. If initial medical therapy fails, then the patient will need to be re-assessed and referred to the appropriate specialist.

There is a significant placebo effect in the treatment of nocturia, and, in general, there is only a small additional decrease in nocturia with active drug therapy, compared to placebo. Accordingly and in view of the manifold aetiologies of nocturia, it seems probable that multiple approaches will be necessary in the majority of patients to achieve benefit to their nocturia which would translate into both improved sleep quality and daytime functioning. Careful objective and subjective documentation of treatment outcomes will hopefully result in future outcomes research allowing for the development of evidence-based guidelines to best practices in the management of patients with nocturia.

4.6.1 **Conclusions**

For a summary of treatments for nocturia, see Tables 4.1 and 4.2.

Table 4.2 Treatment of nocturia by underlying pathology			
Diagnosis	Desmopressin	Antimuscarinics	Alpha-1 blocker
NP	✓		
OAB		✓	
BPO			✓
NP + OAB	✓	✓	
NP + BPO	✓		✓
OAB + BPO		✓	✓
NP + OAB + BPO	✓	✓	✓
BPO, benign prostatic obstruction; NP, nocturnal polyuria; OAB, overactive bladder syndrome.			

References

1. Cho SY, *et al.* Short-term effects of systematized behavioral modification program for nocturia: a prospective study. *Neurourol Urodyn.* 2012;**31**:64–8.

2. Johnson TM 2nd, *et al.* Effects of behavioral and drug therapy on nocturia in older incontinent women. *J Am Geriatr Soc.* 2005;**53**:846–50.

3. Burgio KL, *et al.* Behavioral versus drug treatment for overactive bladder in men: the Male Overactive Bladder Treatment in Veterans (MOTIVE) Trial. *J Am Geriatr Soc.* 2011;**59**:2209–16.

4. Vaughan CP, *et al.* A multicomponent behavioural and drug intervention for nocturia in elderly men: rationale and pilot results. *BJU Int.* 2009;**104**:69–74.

5. Song C, *et al.* Effects of bladder training and/or tolterodine in female patients with overactive bladder syndrome: a prospective, randomized study. *J Korean Med Sci.* 2006;**21**:1060–3.

6. Soda T, *et al.* Efficacy of nondrug lifestyle measures for the treatment of nocturia. *J Urol.* 2010;**184**:1000–4.

7. Tacklind J, *et al.* Finasteride for benign prostatic hyperplasia. *Cochrane Database Syst Rev.* 2010;**10**:CD006015.

8. Johnson TM 2nd, *et al.* The effect of doxazosin, finasteride and combination therapy on nocturia in men with benign prostatic hyperplasia. *J Urol.* 2007;**178**:2045–50; discussion 2050–1.

9. Roehrborn CG, Van Kerrebroeck P, and Nordling J. Safety and efficacy of alfuzosin 10 mg once-daily in the treatment of lower urinary tract symptoms and clinical benign prostatic hyperplasia: a pooled analysis of three double-blind, placebo-controlled studies. *BJU Int.* 2003;**92**:257–61.

10. Zhang K, *et al.* Effect of doxazosin gastrointestinal therapeutic system 4 mg vs tamsulosin 0.2 mg on nocturia in Chinese men with lower urinary tract symptoms: a prospective, multicenter, randomized, open, parallel study. *Urology.* 2011;**78**:636–40.

11. Johnson TM 2nd, *et al.* Changes in nocturia from medical treatment of benign prostatic hyperplasia: secondary analysis of the Department of Veterans Affairs Cooperative Study Trial. *J Urol.* 2003;**170**:145–8.

12. Curran MP. Silodosin: treatment of the signs and symptoms of benign prostatic hyperplasia. *Drugs.* 2011;**71**:897–907.

13. Garimella PS, *et al.* Naftopidil for the treatment of lower urinary tract symptoms compatible with benign prostatic hyperplasia. *Cochrane Database Syst Rev.* 2009;**4**:CD007360.

14. Ukimura O, *et al.* Naftopidil versus tamsulosin hydrochloride for lower urinary tract symptoms associated with benign prostatic hyperplasia with special reference to the storage symptom: a prospective randomized controlled study. *Int J Urol.* 2008;**15**:1049–54.

15. Oh-oka H. Effect of naftopidil on nocturia after failure of tamsulosin. *Urology.* 2008;**72**:1051–5.

16. Vallancien G, *et al.* Alfuzosin 10 mg once daily for treating benign prostatic hyperplasia: a 3-year experience in real-life practice. *BJU Int.* 2008;**101**:847–52.

17. Chapple CR, *et al.* Silodosin therapy for lower urinary tract symptoms in men with suspected benign prostatic hyperplasia: results of an international, randomized, double-blind, placebo- and active-controlled clinical trial performed in Europe. *Eur Urol.* 2011;**59**:342–52.

18. Lojanapiwat B and Permpongkosol S. The efficacy and safety of oral tamsulosin controlled absorption system (OCAS) for the treatment of lower urinary tract symptoms due to bladder outlet obstruction associated with benign prostatic hyperplasia: an open-label preliminary study. *Int Braz J Urol.* 2011;**37**:468–76.

19. Yoshida M, *et al.* Effectiveness of tamsulosin hydrochloride and its mechanism in improving nocturia associated with lower urinary tract symptoms/benign prostatic hyperplasia. *Neurourol Urodyn.* 2010;**29**:1276–81.

20. Yoshida M, *et al.* Effect of tamsulosin hydrochloride on lower urinary tract symptoms and quality of life in patients with benign prostatic hyperplasia. Evaluation using bother score. *Drugs Today (Barc).* 2007;**43** Suppl B:1–7.

21. Abrams P, *et al.* The standardisation of terminology of lower urinary tract function: report from the Standardisation Sub-committee of the International Continence Society. *Neurourol Urodyn.* 2002;**21**:167–78.

22. Roxburgh C, Cook J, and Dublin N. Anticholinergic drugs versus other medications for overactive bladder syndrome in adults. *Cochrane Database Syst Rev.* 2007;**3**:CD003190.

23. Kaplan SA, *et al.* Tolterodine extended release improves overactive bladder symptoms in men with overactive bladder and nocturia. *Urology.* 2006;**68**:328–32.

24. Rackley R, *et al*. Nighttime dosing with tolterodine reduces overactive bladder-related nocturnal micturitions in patients with overactive bladder and nocturia. *Urology*. 2006;**67**:731–6; discussion 736.

25. Wyndaele JJ, *et al*. Effects of flexible-dose fesoterodine on overactive bladder symptoms and treatment satisfaction: an open-label study. *Int J Clin Pract*. 2009;**63**:560–7.

26. Chapple C, *et al*. Clinical efficacy, safety, and tolerability of once-daily fesoterodine in subjects with overactive bladder. *Eur Urol*. 2007;**52**:1204–12.

27. Dmochowski RR, *et al*. Randomized, double-blind, placebo-controlled trial of flexible-dose fesoterodine in subjects with overactive bladder. *Urology*. 2010;**75**:62–8.

28. Herschorn S, *et al*. Comparison of fesoterodine and tolterodine extended release for the treatment of overactive bladder: a head-to-head placebo-controlled trial. *BJU Int*. 2010;**105**:58–66.

29. Nitti VW, *et al*. Efficacy, safety and tolerability of fesoterodine for overactive bladder syndrome. *J Urol*. 2007;**178**:2488–94.

30. Brubaker L and FitzGerald MP. Nocturnal polyuria and nocturia relief in patients treated with solifenacin for overactive bladder symptoms. *Int Urogynecol J Pelvic Floor Dysfunct*. 2007;**18**:737–41.

31. Rudy D, *et al*. Multicenter phase III trial studying trospium chloride in patients with overactive bladder. *Urology*. 2006;**67**:275–80.

32. Zinner N, *et al*. Trospium chloride improves overactive bladder symptoms: a multicenter phase III trial. *J Urol*. 2004;**171**(6 Pt 1):2311–15; quiz 2435.

33. Ginsberg DA, Oefelein MG, and Ellsworth PI. Once-daily administration of trospium chloride extended release provides 24-hr coverage of nocturnal and diurnal symptoms of overactive bladder: an integrated analysis of two phase III trials. *Neurourol Urodyn*. 2011;**30**:563–7.

34. Kaplan SA, *et al*. Tolterodine and tamsulosin for treatment of men with lower urinary tract symptoms and overactive bladder: a randomized controlled trial. *JAMA*. 2006;**296**:2319–28.

35. Yang Y, *et al*. Efficacy and safety of combined therapy with terazosin and tolteradine for patients with lower urinary tract symptoms associated with benign prostatic hyperplasia: a prospective study. *Chin Med J (Engl)*. 2007;**120**:370–4.

36. Kaplan SA, Gonzalez RR, and Te AE. Combination of alfuzosin and sildenafil is superior to monotherapy in treating lower urinary tract symptoms and erectile dysfunction. *Eur Urol*. 2007;**51**:1717–23.

37. van Kerrebroeck P, *et al*. The standardisation of terminology in nocturia: Report from the Standardization Sub-committee of the International Continence Society. *Neurourol Urodyn*. 2002;**21**:179–83.

38. Weiss JP, *et al*. Efficacy and safety of low dose desmopressin orally disintegrating tablet in men with nocturia: results of a multicenter, randomized, double-blind, placebo controlled, parallel group study. *J Urol*. 2013;**190**:965–72.

39. Sand PK, *et al*. Efficacy and safety of low dose desmopressin orally disintegrating tablet in women with nocturia: results of a multicenter, randomized, double-blind, placebo controlled, parallel group study. *J Urol*. 2013;**190**:958–64.

40. Van Kerrebroeck P. Nocturia and Antidiuretic Pharmacotherapy. In: Weiss JP, *et al*. eds. *Nocturia: causes, consequences and clinical approaches*. 2012. Springer Science + Business Media, LLC, pp. 135–44.

41. Zong H, *et al*. Efficacy and safety of desmopressin for treatment of nocturia: a systematic review and meta-analysis of double-blinded trials. *Int Urol Nephrol*. 2012;**44**:377–84.

42. Weiss JP, *et al*. Desmopressin orally disintegrating tablet effectively reduces nocturia: results of a randomized, double-blind, placebo-controlled trial. *Neurourol Urodyn*. 2012;**31**:441–7.

43. Pedersen PA and Johansen PB. Prophylactic treatment of adult nocturia with bumetanide. *Br J Urol*. 1988;**62**:145–7.

44. Reynard JM, *et al*. A novel therapy for nocturnal polyuria: a double-blind randomized trial of frusemide against placebo. *Br J Urol*. 1998;**81**:215–18.

45. Curcio L. *et al*. Use of botulinum toxin type A (Onabotulinum toxin A) through transcystoscopic vesical insertion for overactive bladder syndrome unresponsive to oral medication. *Braz J Video-Sur*. 2008;**1**: 97–103.

46. Hamidi Madani A, *et al*. Transurethral intraprostatic Botulinum toxin-A injection: a novel treatment for BPH refractory to current medical therapy in poor surgical candidates. *World J Urol*. 2013;**31**:235–9.

47. Whelton A. Nephrotoxicity of nonsteroidal anti-inflammatory drugs: physiologic foundations and clinical implications. *Am J Med*. 1999;**106**(5B):13S.

48. Shin HI, *et al*. Long-term effect of loxoprofen sodium on nocturia in patients with benign prostatic hyperplasia. *Korean J Urol*. 2011;**52**:265–8.

49. Falahatkar S, *et al*. Celecoxib for treatment of nocturia caused by benign prostatic hyperplasia: a prospective, randomized, double-blind, placebo-controlled study. *Urology*. 2008;**72**:813–16.

50. Margel D, *et al*. Predictors of nocturia quality of life before and shortly after prostatectomy. *Urology*. 2007;**70**:493–7.

51. Van Dijk MM, *et al*. The role of nocturia in the quality of life of men with lower urinary tract symptoms. *BJU Int*. 2010;**105**:1141–6.

52. Schatzl G, *et al*. The early postoperative morbidity of transurethral resection of the prostate and of 4 minimally invasive treatment alternatives. *J Urol*. 1997;**158**:105–10; discussion 110–11.

53. Simaioforidis V, *et al*. Tamsulosin versus transurethral resection of the prostate: effect on nocturia as a result of benign prostatic hyperplasia. *Int J Urol*. 2011;**18**:243–8.

54. Tacklind J, *et al*. Serenoa repens for benign prostatic hyperplasia. *Cochrane Database Syst Rev*. 2009;**2**:CD001423.

55. Wilt T, *et al*. Pygeum africanum for benign prostatic hyperplasia. *Cochrane Database Syst Rev*. 2002;**1**:CD001044.

56. BarryMJ, *et al*. Effect of increasing doses of saw palmetto extract on lower urinary tract symptoms: a randomized trial. *JAMA*. 2011;**306**:1344–51.

57. Wilt T, *et al*. Cernilton for benign prostatic hyperplasia. *Cochrane Database Syst Rev*. 2000;**2**:CD001042.

58. Kaye M. Nocturia: a blinded, randomized, parallel placebo-controlled self-study of the effect of 5 different sedatives and analgesics. *Can Urol Assoc J*. 2008;**2**:604–8.

59. Vaughan CP, *et al*. A multicomponent behavioural and drug intervention for nocturia in elderly men: rationale and pilot results. *BJU Int*. 2009;**104**:69–74.

60. Drake MJ, Mills IW, and Noble JG. Melatonin pharmacotherapy for nocturia in men with benign prostatic enlargement. *J Urol*. 2004;**171**:1199–202.

61. Sugaya K, *et al*. Effects of melatonin and rilmazafone on nocturia in the elderly. *J Int Med Res*. 2007;**35**:685–91.

Chapter 5

Management of refractory and complex cases of nocturia

David James Osborn, Haerin Lee, and Roger Dmochowski

Key points

- No evidence-based treatments are available for the treatment of refractory or complex nocturia.
- Assessment may involve further investigations such as computed tomography, magnetic resonance imaging, cystoscopy, or urodynamics.
- If nocturia is due to incomplete emptying of the bladder, then treatment options can include intermittent catheterization or long-term urethral or suprapubic catheterization.
- If nocturia is due to an overactive bladder, then treatment options include botulinum toxin A, sacral nerve stimulation, augmentation cystoplasty, or urinary diversion.
- Alternative medicine, such as reflexology, hypnotherapy, and acupuncture, can also be tried.
- Patients need to be made aware that, in refractory and complex cases, none of the treatments have a high level of evidence, and therefore treatment will be individualized according to bothersomeness and effect on quality of life.

5.1 Introduction

This chapter discusses the management of treatment-resistant or complex nocturia that is refractory to lifestyle modifications, behavioural therapy, pharmacotherapy, and endoscopic surgery. Although the prevalence of treatment-resistant nocturia is not known, treatment can be challenging due to this problem's multifactorial aetiology and high variability over time. The goal of management is to improve QoL.

5.2 Patient assessment

Similar to ordinary nocturia, abnormally increased production of urine, decreased bladder capacity, detrusor overactivity, and impaired sleep can all contribute to complex nocturia. Successful treatment of complex cases depends on an accurate assessment of the aetiology; therefore, when a patient has failed traditional management, all non-urological aetiologies must be ruled out. Referral to a sleep medicine specialist and a primary care physician should be considered to assist with a more thorough medical and psychiatric evaluation. Direct communication with other specialties and a multidisciplinary approach may improve the elucidation of an aetiology.

In addition to involving practitioners in other fields to help with diagnosis, axial imaging of the abdomen and pelvis, using computed tomography (CT) scan, is beneficial to rule out uncommon structural and anatomical aetiologies such as a missed distal ureteral stone. In addition, a repeat cystoscopy and urodynamics study should be considered to look for progression of the problem or other entities such as a bladder stone. The initial presentation of undiagnosed neurological conditions, such as multiple sclerosis or central nervous system tumours, may manifest with urological symptoms; therefore, magnetic resonance imaging (MRI) of the head/spine/pelvis for spinal cord or brain lesions could prove helpful.

5.3 Patient management

5.3.1 Once-nightly intermittent catheterization

When a patient's nocturnal urine production is greater than their nocturnal functional bladder capacity, they will need to get up at night to urinate. If a patient voids at night prior to sleep and they completely empty their bladder, their functional bladder capacity is equivalent to the actual bladder capacity. However, if the patient is not able to completely empty their bladder and has a significant PVR volume, they are not taking full advantage of their bladder capacity during the night hours. Therefore, it is reasonable to have the patient perform intermittent catheterization, immediately before going to bed, to assist in emptying the bladder completely, and thereby increase the nocturnal functional bladder capacity without increasing the actual bladder capacity. An increased PVR volume decreases the nocturnal functional bladder capacity by the amount of the PVR.

In 1998, Madersbacher et al. performed a retrospective study of urodynamics in 253 men and 183 women referred to urology for evaluation of LUTS and incontinence, respectively [1]. The researchers found an average PVR of 89 mL in men and 15 mL in women. This significant PVR in men with LUTS was confirmed by another retrospective study in 2001 by Fusco et al., in which the average PVR of 963 men with LUTS was 111 mL [2]. The average PVR in men with nocturia appears to be somewhat lower and ranges from 28 mL to 69 mL in studies of that patient population [3, 4]. Based on the high SD of the mean PVR in all of the studies mentioned, there is significant variation in the ability of patients with nocturia to empty their bladders. Therefore, based on the evidence of increased PVR in the literature, it can be inferred that a significant proportion of patients with nocturia may benefit from once-nightly intermittent catheterization.

Though there are no studies of the effect of once-nightly intermittent catheterization on nocturia, there are multiple studies that show the benefit of intermittent catheterization on symptoms related to nocturia. Both Pilloni et al. and Kessler et al. published their results of the beneficial effects of intermittent catheterization in adults with nocturia [5, 6]. In the Kessler study, the average frequency of catheterization was three times per day, and, in the Pilloni study, the range of catheterization frequency was 1–5 times per day and the infection rate was 0.84 per year per patient. Sixty per cent or more of included patients experienced substantial improvement in QoL in both trials.

With this type of treatment, infection is one of the biggest concerns. Clearly, once-nightly catheterization will increase a patient's risk of a urinary tract infection because of the introduction of small amounts of bacteria into a bladder that is not completely emptying. To reduce this risk, a new catheter can be used every time, or a sterile, instead of a clean, technique can be used [7]. For men, hydrophilic catheters may be more comfortable and decrease the risk of infection, compared to traditional plastic catheters [8].

In men, an alternative is to have a urinal bottle by the bedside, into which to void at night if they have difficulty walking to the toilet or do not want to walk to the toilet.

5.3.2 Indwelling catheter

For patients with OAB that results in incontinence, AUA guidelines do not recommend a chronic indwelling catheter [9]. This section of the AUA guideline is based on expert opinion and does not mention the treatment of OAB with nocturia as the primary symptom. It is this opinion of the authors of this chapter that chronic transurethral catheterization is not recommended and will not improve the QoL of patients with nocturia. Long-term transurethral catheterization can result in iatrogenic injury to the urethra, epididymitis, pyelonephritis, bladder stones, kidney or ureteral stones, and damage to the upper urinary tract. The rates of these complications are lower with a suprapubic catheter, compared to a transurethral catheter [10].

In a patient who has severe nocturia as a result of nocturnal polyuria or a small-capacity bladder and when all other treatment options have failed, a suprapubic catheter may improve QoL. Though there are no studies looking at the use of a suprapubic catheter in patients with OAB, there is recent evidence in the literature that shows this form of bladder drainage may have fewer complications than previously published and improve QoL in patients with spinal cord injury [11].

Although the authors of this chapter have never placed a suprapubic tube for the sole indication of nocturia, a temporary Foley catheter, placed at night and removed by the patient on a daily basis, has been recommended to a select group of patients. This treatment would work best for patients with a limited bladder capacity or nocturnal polyuria. Whilst this form of treatment most likely has a lower rate of complications than a chronic indwelling catheter, the risk of infection and discomfort is significant. The use of an indwelling catheter, in conjunction with onabotulinum toxin A, whilst not optimal, may be a useful strategy for those subjects unwilling to perform intermittent catheterization.

5.3.3 Intradetrusor onabotulinum toxin A

In January 2013, the FDA approved onabotulinum toxin A for use in patients with non-neurogenic, medication-refractory OAB. In August 2013, Chapple *et al.* published their results of a randomized, double-blind, placebo-controlled trial of intradetrusor onabotulinum toxin A for patients with idiopathic OAB symptoms [12]. The researchers found that this form of treatment significantly improved the number of nocturia episodes, compared to placebo (decrease of 0.36 episodes per night). Interestingly, this change was ten times less significant than the improvement in other symptoms of OAB such as urgency incontinence and urinary frequency. This might indicate that onabotulinum toxin A is not as effective for treating nocturia as it is for the other symptoms of OAB. In addition, if nocturnal polyuria is the predominant cause of nocturia, onabotulinum toxin A would be an even less effective option.

However, there may be some utility in using high dosages of onabotulinum toxin A in select patients with severe nocturia. In these patients, paralysis of the bladder with onabotulinum toxin A dosages as high as 300 units, in conjunction with clean intermittent catheterization, at least four times per day, may improve QoL of life. In 2009, Kessler *et al.* published their results showing an improvement in QoL of patients who went into urinary retention and required intermittent catheterization after intradetrusor onabotulinum toxin A injection for non-neurogenic OAB [13].

5.3.4 Nerve stimulation

Neuromodulation is a surgical option for complex treatment-refractory nocturia. The two modalities most commonly used are sacral nerve stimulation (SNS) and percutaneous posterior tibial nerve stimulation (PTNS). Currently, according to FDA and AUA guidelines, SNS is approved as the third-line treatment of non-neurogenic OAB. Similar to other treatment modalities discussed in this chapter, there is little evidence in the literature to support the use of SNS in patients with the prevailing symptom of nocturia.

The authors of the AUA guidelines reviewed the current literature pertaining to SNS and found that, in general, all 13 quality studies in the literature showed improvement in urgency incontinence and symptoms of OAB [9]. Interestingly, however, very few of those studies comment specifically on nocturia. In one of the studies that did mention nocturia, Sutherland et al. showed a statistically significant improvement of one void per night in a retrospective review of 104 patients who underwent SNS [14]. Even after including a few studies that show improvement in nocturia in patients with interstitial cystitis after SNS, the evidence to support the use of SNS in patients with the symptom of nocturia is surprisingly lacking [15, 16]. However, this is still a treatment that should be considered in a patient with severe nocturia that has failed all other less invasive forms of treatment.

Unlike SNS, PTNS has more data in the literature to support its use in patients with nocturia. One of the first studies that commented on the effect of PTNS on nocturia was a 2001 multi-centre trial of 53 patients by Govier et al. [17]. In that study, post-PTNS 3-day voiding diaries showed that PTNS was well tolerated and reduced night-time voids in patients with OAB by 21%. A 2009 RCT of 100 patients found similarly that PTNS was safe and effective for OAB, with objective outcomes comparable to those of pharmacotherapy [18]. In that trial, nocturia decreased by an average of 0.7 voids per night in the treatment group. One year later, a larger trial of 220 patients compared PTNS to a sham treatment [19]. That study showed that, when compared to a sham treatment, PTNS improved OAB symptoms and decreased night-time voids by an average of 0.7 times per night. PTNS therefore may be an excellent minimally invasive option, given its efficacy in treating urinary tract symptoms, without requiring the placement of a permanent implant. Limitations include cost, frequency of office visits, and the need to continue maintenance therapy beyond the initial 12 weeks of therapy.

5.3.5 **Bladder augmentation (enterocystoplasty)**

There are no studies in the literature that describe enterocystoplasty for nocturia; however, there are a few relatively recent studies that describe the outcomes of this surgery for benign disease, including refractory OAB. In one of these studies from 2005 presenting the outcomes of 76 patients who underwent bladder augmentation for benign disease, 12% of patients had the surgery performed for the indication of refractory OAB [20]. All 12 patients were clinically cured or improved after the surgery. In another earlier study from 1998, Awad et al. looked at their results of bladder augmentation in 51 women with refractory urgency incontinence and found that 78% of patients were continent or had only occasional leakage [21]. Interestingly, 39% of patients required intermittent catheterization to empty their bladder. After enterocystoplasty, patients must be willing to perform intermittent catheterization to aid in bladder emptying and to possibly irrigate the bladder to decrease the risk of infection and stone formation. An enterocystoplasty, combined with a supratrigonal cystectomy, has been described in the literature as a treatment for patients with interstitial cystitis; however, this surgical technique is clearly not indicated in patients with nocturia [22].

Twenty years ago, bladder augmentation was one of the few treatment options for refractory OAB symptoms, and both of the studies mentioned present data from surgeries performed decades earlier (between 1987 and 1993). Although the authors of this chapter have never performed bladder augmentation for this indication, it may improve the QoL in the very select patients with severe nocturia, but there is little evidence to support this in the literature. In addition, there are significant perioperative complications such as blood transfusion, pneumonia, and myocardial infarction. Even further, there are numerous long-term complications of this major surgery such as kidney stone disease, chronic diarrhoea, pyelonephritis, and malignancy [23].

5.3.6 **Urinary diversion**

Similar to a bladder augmentation, simple cystectomies are rarely performed for benign disease, and the literature supporting this treatment option is sparse for non-neurogenic OAB, and non-existent for the indication of nocturia. In 2011, Rowley *et al.* presented their results of supratrigonal simple cystectomies with urinary diversion performed on 23 patients with benign disease [24]. In this study, there were four patients who had their bladders removed for the indication of incontinence; however, there was no comment about any of the patients having OAB symptoms. Nine patients had post-operative complications, ranging from two superficial wound infections to a pulmonary embolus and a fascial dehiscence. The AUA guidelines state that, based on expert opinion, urinary diversion can be used to treat patients with refractory, complicated OAB; however, no mention is made of patients with severe nocturia as the predominant symptom.

In 1997, Singh *et al.* published their results of urinary diversion without a cystectomy in patients with benign disease [25]. In this study, only three of the 93 patients underwent urinary diversion for non-neurogenic OAB, and no comment was made about nocturia. Although it is technically easier not to remove the bladder, this study reports an unacceptably high 52% rate of recurrent vesical infection and pyocystis. There are several other articles in the literature that also describe a high rate of pyocystis when the bladder is not removed [26, 27]. It does not appear that urinary diversion without supratrigonal cystectomy is an acceptable treatment option for nocturia.

5.3.7 **Alternative medicine**

Although the quality of the literature in the area of alternative medicine is variable, it may be possible to treat refractory nocturia with alternative medicine treatments such as acupuncture, hypnosis, and reflexology.

5.3.7.1 *Acupuncture*

There is sparse evidence in the literature supporting the use of acupuncture in patients with nocturia; however, there are a few more studies that support its use in patients with OAB or insomnia. In 2002, Nadia Ellis performed a small placebo-controlled study of acupuncture in elderly patients with nocturia and concluded that the 11 patients in the treatment arm had a clinically significant reduction in nocturia, compared to the nine patients in the placebo arm [28]. In a later much larger randomized, placebo-controlled trial of 85 patients with OAB from 2005, there was a significant difference in outcomes between acupuncture needles placed in the proper location and those placed at a sham location [29]. In this study, even though both groups showed improvement, the treatment group showed significantly more improvement in subjective symptoms of OAB and bladder capacity, compared to the placebo group.

In a study from 2002, Tanaka *et al.* manipulated acupuncture needles inserted into the periosteum of the sacrum in anaesthetized rats [30]. The authors concluded that this technique resulted in a suppression of bladder activity and a stimulation of brain activity on the electroencephalogram (EEG), similar to sleep. There is also evidence in humans that acupuncture might improve sleep. In their review of literature from November 2001 to January 2003, Sok *et al.* found that there is support in the literature to suggest that acupuncture might be an effective treatment option for patients with insomnia [31].

Although more research is needed, both studies on insomnia and OAB support the statement that acupuncture may be beneficial in some patients with refractory nocturia.

5.3.7.2 *Hypnosis*

In contrast to acupuncture, there are only scattered case reports in the literature that purport the benefits of hypnosis for OAB, and no description of its use in patients with refractory nocturia.

5.3.7.3 Reflexology

In the only large study that examines the effect of reflexology (massaging of pressure points on the feet) on OAB, Mak et al. performed an RCT comparing reflexology to foot massage in 120 women with OAB [32]. In this study, the authors concluded that reflexology showed a significant improvement in daytime urinary frequency, compared to foot massage. Clearly, more research is needed in this area before any conclusions can be drawn about the efficacy of reflexology for nocturia or any other form of OAB.

5.4 Conclusions

The evidence to support different treatment modalities for refractory and complex cases of nocturia in the literature is sparse, and the majority of evidence in this chapter is drawn from studies that examine patients with refractory OAB, and not specifically nocturia. The use of invasive treatment options, such as enterocystoplasty or urinary diversion, for patients with refractory nocturia is not supported by the literature, and the discussion is based on extrapolation from the use of these surgeries in patients with mixed OAB symptoms. If a non-reversible therapy is considered, it is advisable to involve multiple physicians in the decision-making process and consider a referral to a tertiary medical centre.

References

1. Madersbacher S, et al. The aging lower urinary tract: a comparative urodynamic study of men and women. Urology. 1998;**51**:206–12.

2. Fusco F, et al. Videourodynamic studies in men with lower urinary tract symptoms: a comparison of community based versus referral urological practices. J Urol. 2001;**166**:910–13.

3. Drake MJ, Mills IW, and Noble JG.: Melatonin pharmacotherapy for nocturia in men with benign prostatic enlargement. J Urol. 2004;**171**:1199–202.

4. Johnson TM, et al. The effect of doxazosin, finasteride and combination therapy on nocturia in men with benign prostatic hyperplasia. J Urol. 2007;**178**:2045–50;discussion 2050–1.

5. Pilloni S, et al. Intermittent catheterisation in older people: a valuable alternative to an indwelling catheter? Age Ageing. 2005;**34**:57–60.

6. Kessler TM, Ryu G, and Burkhard FC. Clean intermittent self-catheterization: a burden for the patient? Neurourol Urodyn. 2009;**28**:18–21.

7. Hudson E and Murahata RI. The 'no-touch' method of intermittent urinary catheter insertion: can it reduce the risk of bacteria entering the bladder? Spinal Cord. 2005;**43**:611–14.

8. Vapnek JM, Maynard FM, and Kim J. A prospective randomized trial of the LoFric hydrophilic coated catheter versus conventional plastic catheter for clean intermittent catheterization. J Urol. 2003;**169**:994–8.

9. Gormley EA, et al. Diagnosis and treatment of overactive bladder (non-neurogenic) in adults: AUA/SUFU guideline. Available at: <http://www.auanet.org/common/pdf/education/clinical-guidance/Overactive-Bladder.pdf> (accessed 30 September, 2013).

10. Weld KJ and Dmochowski RR. Effect of bladder management on urological complications in spinal cord injured patients. J Urol. 2000;**163**:768–72.

11. Feifer A and Corcos J. Contemporary role of suprapubic cystostomy in treatment of neuropathic bladder dysfunction in spinal cord injured patients. Neurourol Urodyn. 2008;**27**:475–9.

12. Chapple C, Sievert K-D, Macdiarmid S, et al. Onabotulinum toxin A 100 U Significantly improves all idiopathic overactive bladder symptoms and quality of life in patients with overactive bladder and urinary incontinence. A randomised, double-blind, placebo-controlled trial. Eur Urol. 2013;**64**:249–56.

13. Kessler TM, et al. Clean intermittent self-catheterization after botulinum neurotoxin type A injections: short-term effect on quality of life. Obstet Gynecol. 2009;**113**:1046–51.

14. Sutherland SE, et al. Sacral nerve stimulation for voiding dysfunction: one institution's 11-year experience. Neurourol Urodyn. 2007;**26**:19–28; discussion 36.

15. Maher CF, *et al*. Percutaneous sacral nerve root neuromodulation for intractable interstitial cystitis. *J Urol*. 2001;**165**:884–6.

16. Comiter CV. Sacral neuromodulation for the symptomatic treatment of refractory interstitial cystitis: a prospective study. *J Urol*. 2003;**169**:1369–73.

17. Govier FE, *et al*. Percutaneous afferent neuromodulation for the refractory overactive bladder: results of a multicenter study. *J Urol*. 2001;**165**:1193–8.

18. Peters KM, *et al*. Randomized trial of percutaneous tibial nerve stimulation versus extended-release tolterodine: results from the overactive bladder innovative therapy trial. *J Urol*. 2009;**182**:1055–61.

19. Peters KM, *et al*. Randomized trial of percutaneous tibial nerve stimulation versus sham efficacy in the treatment of overactive bladder syndrome: results from the SUmiT trial. *J Urol*. 2010;**183**:1438–43.

20. Blaivas JG, *et al*. Long-term followup of augmentation enterocystoplasty and continent diversion in patients with benign disease. *J Urol*. 2005;**173**:1631–4.

21. Awad SA, *et al*. Long-term results and complications of augmentation ileocystoplasty for idiopathic urge incontinence in women. *Br J Urol*. 1998;**81**:569–73.

22. Peeker R, Aldenborg F, and Fall M. The treatment of interstitial cystitis with supratrigonal cystectomy and ileocystoplasty: difference in outcome between classic and nonulcer disease. *J Urol*. 1998;**159**:1479–82.

23. Gilbert SM and Hensle TW. Metabolic consequences and long-term complications of enterocystoplasty in children: a review. *J Urol*. 2005;**173**:1080–6.

24. Rowley MW, *et al*. Simple cystectomy: outcomes of a new operative technique. *Urology*. 2011;**78**:942–5.

25. Singh G, Wilkinson JM, and Thomas DG. Supravesical diversion for incontinence: a long-term follow-up. *Br J Urol*. 1997;**79**:348–53.

26. Fazili T, B*et al*. Fate of the leftover bladder after supravesical urinary diversion for benign disease. *J Urol*. 2006;**176**:620–1.

27. Kato H, *et al*. Fate of tetraplegic patients managed by ileal conduit for urinary control: long-term follow-up. *Int J Urol*. 2002;**9**:253–6.

28. Ellis N. A pilot study to evaluate the effect of acupuncture on nocturia in the elderly. *Complement Ther Med*. 1993;**1**:164–7.

29. Emmons SL and Otto L. Acupuncture for overactive bladder: a randomized controlled trial. *Obstet Gynecol*. 2005;**106**:138–3.

30. Tanaka Y, *et al*. Effects of acupuncture to the sacral segment on the bladder activity and electroencephalogram. *Psychiatry Clin Neurosci*. 2002;**56**:249–50.

31. Sok SR, Erlen JA, and Kim KB. Effects of acupuncture therapy on insomnia. *J Adv Nurs*. 2003;**44**:375–84.

32. Mak H-LJ, *et al*. Randomized controlled trial of foot reflexology for patients with symptomatic idiopathic detrusor overactivity. *Int Urogynecol J Pelvic Floor Dysfunct*. 2007;**18**:653–8.

Chapter 6

Guidelines

Hashim Hashim and Paul Abrams

Key points
• No established or agreed guidelines or algorithms are available.
• The International Continence Society published a basic algorithm in 2002 for the management of nocturia [1].
• In 2010, the Committee for Establishment of the Clinical Guidelines for Nocturia of the Neurogenic Bladder Society published an algorithm for the treatment of nocturia [2].
• In 2013, the International Consultation on Urological Diseases included an algorithm for the treatment of nocturia in men [3].
• We have devised a treatment algorithm (figure 6.1), which incorporates information from all the above guidelines.

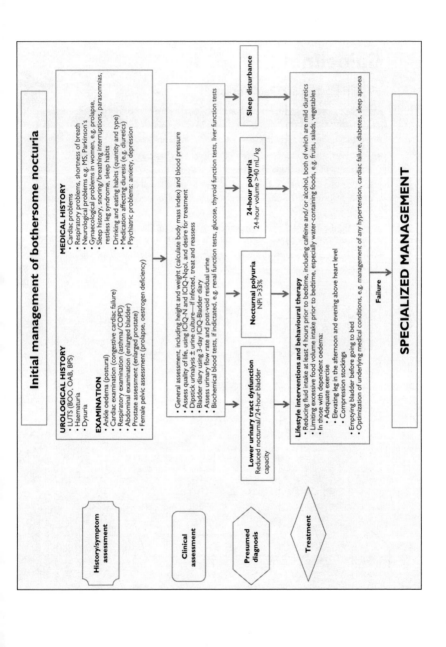

Initial management of bothersome nocturia

History/symptom assessment

UROLOGICAL HISTORY
- LUTS (BOO, OAB, BPS)
- Haematuria
- Dysuria

EXAMINATION
- Ankle oedema (postural)
- Cardiac examination (congestive cardiac failure)
- Respiratory examination (asthma/COPD)
- Abdominal examination (enlarged bladder)
- Prostate assessment (enlarged prostate)
- Female pelvic assessment (prolapse, oestrogen deficiency)

MEDICAL HISTORY
- Cardiac problems
- Respiratory problems, shortness of breath
- Neurological problems e.g. MS, Parkinson's
- Gynaecological problems in women, e.g. prolapse,
- Sleep history, snoring/breathing interruptions, parasomnias, restless leg syndrome, sleep habits
- Drinking and eating habits (quantity and type)
- Medication affecting diuresis (e.g. diuretics)
- Psychiatric problems: anxiety, depression

Clinical assessment

- General assessment, including height and weight (calculate body mass index) and blood pressure
- Assess quality of life, using ICIQ-N and ICIQ-Nqol, and desire for treatment
- Dipstick urinalysis ± urine culture—if infected, treat and reassess
- Bladder diary using 3-day ICIQ-Bladder diary
- Assess urinary flow rate and post-void residual urine
- Biochemical blood tests, if indictated, e.g. renal function tests, glucose, thyroid function tests, liver function tests

Presumed diagnosis

| Lower urinary tract dysfunction
Reduced nocturnal/24-hour bladder capacity | Nocturnal polyuria
NPi >33% | 24-hour polyuria
24-hour volume >40 mL/kg | Sleep disturbance |

Treatment

Lifestyle interventions and behavioural therapy
- Reducing fluid intake at least 4 hours prior to bedtime, including caffeine and/or alcohol, both of which are mild diuretics
- Limiting excessive food volume intake prior to bedtime, especially water-containing foods, e.g. fruits, salads, vegetables
- In those with dependent oedema:
  - Adequate exercise
  - Elevating leg in the afternoon and evening above heart level
  - Compression stockings
- Emptying bladder before going to bed
- Optimization of underlying medical conditions, e.g. management of any hypertension, cardiac failure, diabetes, sleep apnoea

Failure

SPECIALIZED MANAGEMENT

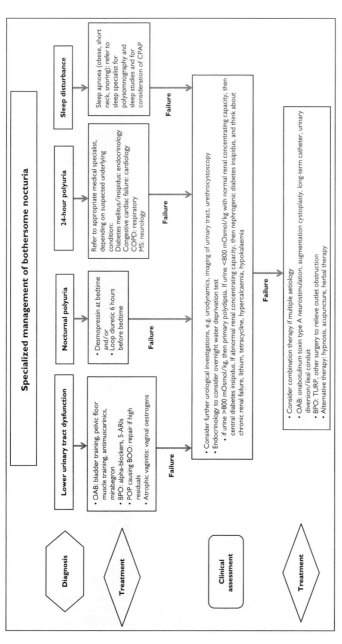

Figure 6.1 Algorithm for the initial and specialized management of bothersome nocturia. 5-ARI, 5-alpha reductase inhibitor; BOO, bladder outlet obstruction; BPO, benign prostatic obstruction; BPS, bladder pain syndrome; COPD, chronic obstructive pulmonary disease; CPAP, continuous positive airway pressure; LUTS, lower urinary tract symptom; MS, multiple sclerosis; OAB, overactive bladder syndrome; POP, pelvic organ prolapse; TURP, transurethral resection of prostate.

Data from: van Kerrebroeck P, et al. The standardisation of terminology in nocturia: report from the Standardisation Sub-committee of the International Continence Society. *Neurourol Urodyn.* 2002;**21**(2):179–83; The Committee for Establishment of the Clinical Guidelines for Nocturia of the Neurogenic Bladder Society. Clinical guidelines for nocturia. *Int J Urol.* 2010;**17**(5):397–409; Chapple C, Abrams P. *Male Lower Urinary Tract Symptoms (LUTS).* Montreal, Canada: Société Internationale d'Urologie (SIU); 2013. pp. 536–537.

References

1. van Kerrebroeck P, *et al*. The standardisation of terminology in nocturia: report from the Standardisation Sub-committee of the International Continence Society. *Neurourol Urodyn*. 2002;**21**:179–83.

2. Committee for Establishment of the Clinical Guidelines for Nocturia of the Neurogenic Bladder Society. Clinical guidelines for nocturia. *Int J Urol*. 2010;**17**:397–409.

3. Chapple C and Abrams P. *Male Lower Urinary Tract Symptoms (LUTS)*. 2013. Montreal: Société Internationale d'Urologie (SIU), pp. 536–7.

Index